Whole Foods Diet Cookbook 2-in-1:

Instant Pot Recipes

&

Meal Prep with Oven-Baked Recipes

ISBN-13: 978-1986049047

ISBN-10: 1986049043

Subject include: whole food cookbooks, whole food diet, meal prep, meal prep cookbook, healthy meal prep cookbook, meal prep for beginners, whole 30, whole 30 diet, whole 30 cookbook, whole 30 diet recipes, whole 30 diet cookbook

Table of Contents

Introduction *12*

Benefits of the Whole Foods Diet Plan *14*

Foods to Eat *16*

Foods to Avoid *18*

Your Healthy Living *20*

Home Cooking with Your Instant Pot *23*

Soup Recipes *25*

   Chicken Soup with Veggies and Mushrooms *26*

   Quick and Easy Tomato Soup *28*

   Savory Beet Soup *30*

   Veggie Soup with Mushrooms *32*

   Lentil Soup without Meat *34*

   Creamy Artichoke Soup *36*

   Cabbage Roll Soup *38*

   Brazilian Shrimp Soup *39*

   Cuban Black Bean Soup *41*

   Easy Mushroom Soup with Barley *43*

   Chicken Meatball Soup *44*

   Celery Potato Soup *46*

   Navy Bean Soup with Bacon *48*

   Quick Onion Soup *50*

   Carrot Soup with Ginger *51*

   Beef & Barley Soup *53*

   Fresh Corn Chowder with Bacon *55*

Stuffed Cabbage Soup *57*

Cajun Style Fish Soup *59*

Asparagus Soup with Ham *61*

Vegetarian Recipes *62*

Barley and Mushrooms Risotto *63*

Quick & Healthy Brussels Sprouts *65*

African Spinach Stew *66*

Green Beans & Tofu Salad *68*

Bulgur Salad with Oranges and Almonds *69*

Black Bean & Quinoa Chili *71*

Israeli Couscous *73*

Spicy Pinto Beans *74*

Feta Wheat Berry Salad *75*

Garlic Chickpeas *77*

Quinoa with Feta & Tomatoes *78*

Mashed Butternut Squash and Apples *80*

Delicious Barley Salad *81*

Sauteed Red Cabbage *82*

Tasty Vegetable Oats *83*

Pumpkin Porridge *85*

Potato Salad with Green Beans *86*

Carried Lentils & Tomato Sauce *88*

Creamy & Light Mashed Sweet Potatoes *89*

Lentil Vegetable Salad *90*

Indian Style Cauliflower with Potatoes *92*

New Potatoes with Garlic and Herbs *94*

Sweet Potato & Kale Stew 95

Creamy Mushroom Risotto 97

Vegetarian Lemon Risotto 99

Rice Pudding with Honey 101

Mexican Style Rice 103

Vegan Stew with Mushrooms 104

Persian Split Pea Stew 106

Egg Recipes 108

Easy Peeled Hard Boiled Eggs 109

Deviled Eggs 110

Cheesy Egg Bake 111

Poultry Recipes 113

Whole Roasted Chicken 114

Chicken with Brown Rice 115

Simple Shredded Chicken 117

Turkey Meatballs in Tomato Sauce 118

Asian Orange Chicken 120

Buffalo Chicken with Potatoes 121

Cheesy Lemon Chicken 122

Duck with Mushrooms and Sweet Onions 123

Barbecue Chili Chicken 125

Turkey Breast with Gravy 126

Chicken Tacos with Chipotles 128

Turkey One Pot Meal 130

Braised Duck with Potatoes 132

Fish & Seafood Recipes 134

Salmon with Broccoli & Potatoes..135

Halibut with Tomatoes, Olives & Capers............................136

Spicy Lemon Salmon..138

Cod with Ginger & Broccoli..139

Shrimp Bisque 140

Shrimp Scampi 142

Shrimp & Potato Stew...143

Mustard Trout Fillets..145

Mediterranean Style Cod 146

Chinese Style Tilapia...147

Pork Recipes 148

Pork Chops with Mashed Potatoes............................149

Pork & Green Chili Stew 151

Pork Roast with Mushroom Gravy 153

Pork Loin with Apples & Cherries............................155

Quick Pork & Rice...156

Chipotle Pork Carnitas 158

Milk-braised Pork 160

Pork Teriyaki..161

Italian Style Pork Ragu 163

Delicious Pork Stew 165

Beef Recipes..167

Quick Beef Meatballs...168

Korean Beef...169

Beef & Rice Stuffed Peppers.......................................171

Mediterranean Beef 173

Spicy Braised Beef...175

Marinated Steak 177

Roast Beef & Carrots 178

Beef Stroganoff 179

Lamb Recipes 181

Lamb Curry...182

Moroccan Style Lamb Stew with Dates & Cinnamon 184

Irish Lamb Stew 186

Conclusion...188

Meal Prep with Oven-Baked Recipes..........................189

Introduction 190

Benefits of Meal Prep 192

Food Prep Containers..195

Your Meal Plan and Grocery List.....................................196

Shopping & Storing 199

Food Prep 201

Poultry Recipes...202

Chicken Rice & Veggie Bowl..204

Healthy Chicken Fajita with Brown Rice...........................206

Honey-Lime Chicken with Sweet Potatoes & Asparagus 208

Chicken Mozzarella Pasta with Tomato Sauce 210

BBQ Chicken Drumsticks and Spaghetti Squash 212

Buffalo Chicken Casserole 214

Chicken Pizza..216

Chicken Enchilada Bowl..217

Pan-roasted Chicken with Couscous and Arugula............219

Garlic Parmesan Chicken Tenders with Green Beans 221

Creamy Garlic Chicken Zucchini Noodles 223

Easy Chicken & Asparagus Sheet Pan 224

Chicken Curry and Couscous 225

Chipotle Shredded Chicken with Cilantro Slaw 227

Chicken Tuscan Pasta Bake 229

Moroccan Chicken with Veggies and Lemon Couscous ...231

Roasted Chicken and Veggies with Miso-Honey Butter ..233

Teriyaki Chicken with Rice and Veggies 235

Chicken Shawarma with Sweet Potato Fry 237

Greek Chicken with Quinoa and Cucumber Salad 239

Easy Jerk Chicken 241

Chicken Butternut Squash Pasta 242

Italian Chicken Bowls 244

Chicken in Peanut Lemon Sauce 246

Ground Turkey Taco Bowls 248

Thai Basil Ground Turkey 250

Turkey Burgers & Sweet Potato Fries 252

Roasted Turkey Breast & Vegetables 254

Egg Recipes 256

Scrambled Eggs with Turmeric 258

Sausage Hash Brown Casserole 259

Veggie Egg Muffins 260

Healthy Breakfast Pizza 262

Breakfast Stuffed Bell Peppers 264

Seafood Recipes 266

Roasted Salmon with Vegetables 268

Salmon Fajita..270

Salmon with Bok Choy and Mushrooms 271

Salmon with Potatoes and Riced Cauliflower 273

Garlic Ginger Basil Salmon 274

Tuna, Veggie and Quinoa Salad 276

Tuna Poke Bowl 277

Creamy Tuna Noodle Casserole.......................................278

Fish Taco Quinoa Bowls 280

Sheet Pan Cod with Mushrooms and Onion 282

Chinese Style Baked Cod 283

One Pan Baked Cod with Vegetables 284

Sheet Pan Pineapple Shrimp with Bell Peppers 285

Shrimp & Chickpea Pasta 286

Shrimp, Veggies, and Cauliflower Rice 288

Shrimp and Cilantro-Lime Quinoa Bowl 289

Halibut with Peach and Pepper Salsa...............................291

Pan-Fried Trout with Tomato Basil Sauce 293

Tilapia in Coconut-Curry Sauce.......................................294

Baked Tilapia with Garlic Breadcrumbs...........................296

Beef Recipes..297

Chipotle and Paprika Eye Round Roast.............................299

Beef and Zucchini Noodles Lasagna 301

Steak Bites 303

Quick and Easy Meatballs 304

Beef Burgers with Vegetables..305

One Pot Salsa Beef Skillet 306

Bleu Cheese Petit Sirloin 308

One Pot Steak & Potatoes 310

Korean Ground Beef and Brown Rice Bowls 311

Stuffed Mexican-Style Bell Peppers 313

Pork Recipes 315

Pork Chop Ranch Sheet Pan 317

Herb-Crusted Pork Chops 319

Balsamic Pork Chops with Peppers 321

Molasses-Orange Pork Chops with Skillet-Roasted Sweet Potatoes 322

Pork Cutlets with Beans and Bell Peppers 324

Dijon Pork with Fruits and Quinoa 326

Ginger Pork Lettuce Wraps 327

Pork Tenderloin with Carrots and Potatoes 329

Spicy Pulled Pork 330

BBQ Pulled Pork Bowls 332

Creamy Pulled Pork Pasta 334

Veggie, Lentil & Whole Grain Recipes 336

Lentil Bowl with Feta and Veggies 338

Sesame-Ginger Fried Rice 340

Simple Tofu Scramble Breakfast 342

One Pot Black Bean & Pumpkin Chili 344

Creamy Butternut Squash Pasta with Mushrooms 346

Chickpea and Lentil Curry 348

Burrito Bowl with Black Beans 350

Lentil Salad with Olives and Cucumbers 351

Lentil Shepherd's Pie with Mushrooms and Sweet Potatoes 353

Honey-Roasted Brussels Sprouts with Lentil-Quinoa Pilaf 355

Turkish-Style White Beans Salad 357

Lentil Bolognese Pasta 359

Thai-Style Quinoa Salad with Lime Vinaigrette 361

Polenta Bowls with Caramelized Onions and Kale 363

Vegetable Enchilada 364

Orange Ginger Tofu 366

Simple Vegetable Fried Rice 368

Healthy Ramen Noodle Salad 370

Baked Sticky Sesame Cauliflower 372

Greek-Style Kale Salad with Feta 374

Wild Rice with Beets and Pecans 376

Snack and Dessert Recipes 378

Blueberry Pancake Bites 380

Healthy Energy Bars 382

Banana Coconut Cookies 383

Sweet Energy Bites 384

Multi-Seed Crackers 385

Conclusion 387

Introduction

First of all, I want to thank you for choosing this book. This cookbook focuses on the whole foods recipes, which provide your body with a numerous health benefits. This diet strategy can be extremely efficient if you manage to follow it sedulously. Apparently, you shouldn't leave it half way through; give yourself at least three weeks of the whole foods nutrition.

In order to make your start more manageable, I have collected many recipes for you. I have also tried to use easily available and budget-friendly ingredients. In general, any foods that unprocessed, unrefined and free from chemicals and preservatives will count as whole foods. The diet is a plant-based so that you will eat lots of fruits, vegetables, whole grains, nuts, legumes, seed, and herbs. Also, you are allowed to eat moderate portions of meat, seafood, and eggs. Choose foods with very few ingredients and all recognizable ingredients.

Avoid anything with more than six ingredients or foods made with ingredients you cannot pronounce. Don't buy frozen meals, canned foods, and drinks. Some snacks are labeled as health food, but generally, they are not healthy at all. It's just a next marketing trick from the company-producer.

Eating whole foods in their most nutritious form provide you with all necessary vitamins, minerals, and other vital nutrients. Antioxidants protect your cells against damage and degeneration. That's why people notice a significant change in their overall wellbeing after shifting to the whole foods eating plan. You will get better teeth and nail health. And your hair will be stronger and shinier, so you'll forget about split ends and hair fall.

Probably the most curious thing about various 30-day diet schemes is that there is no substantial scientific evidence behind most of them. The same way, many people believe that new habit can be formed just in 21 days. In his work on self-image, Dr. Maxwell Maltz wrote that his patients needed about three weeks to adjust to the new situation. Dr. Maltz was a plastic surgeon; his book became a real bestseller, and as a result, now 21-30-day timelines are quoted as some statistical facts. The studies on this subject show that it takes from 2 to 8 months to build a new habit. And still, I suppose that 30-day challenge is a good start. This time framework is long enough to notice positive changes and short enough to be inspiring.

Fruits and veggies fill our bodies with energy in a most natural way. That means the consistent energy flow during the day without undesired peaks and drops of your energy levels. You will feel incredibly energetic even at the end of day's work. Whole foods are full of brain-healthy ingredients that will increase the level of serotonin and cut down cortisol. As a result, you will experience less distress and anxiety.

It's a well-known fact that with time junk food could impact the people's taste. On the flip side, consuming whole foods helps to appreciate the natural taste of the meals. Also, it will be easier for you to eat within your limit. When you eat foods that free from chemicals and processing, you don't tend to overeat. So, weight loss is another positive side effect of the diet.

Eating foods that are rich in fiber increases your digestive capacity. You won't feel heavy after your meals. The food will easily digest and pass through without getting stuck in your system. Your liver and gut will smoothly function so you will have a chance to improve your metabolism and even enhance your immunity. Did you know that our digestive tract contains 70% of our immune defenses?

Nutrient density is an essential factor in making healthy food choices. The whole foods diet is rich in vitamin E and other nutrients that enhance your hair-nails-teeth health. As a result, you'll get healthy and shiny hair. Also, you'll be able to grow your nails long and have lesser dental complaints.

Your ability to think clearly will improve through the consumption of whole foods. This effect will enhance your confidence and increase your productivity. That's right, healthy eating and confidence go hand in hand. And as we know, confident people tend to set new goals, improve physical shape, and maintain good general health along the way.

You shouldn't count each and every calorie you eat. In fact, recipes from this book don't even contain information about calorie content. Most of us are absolutely terrible at calorie reporting. Only small minority of people is willing to measure and weigh everything they eat. And the more overweight you are, the worse you are likely to be at tracking your portion sizes and estimating how many calories you ingest. Surely, calorie-counting can be helpful in the short term. However, in the long term, this approach leads to weight regain after the diet ends. Instead, Whole foods diet offers your body the tools to manage your appetite and help you lose weight more effectively.

Whole foods generally include plant-based foods such as fruits, veggies, seeds and nuts, and animal foods such as poultry, eggs, meat, and seafood. In other words, if it's farmed, fished, hunted or grows in the ground, you can consume it.

Eat all kinds of fresh vegetables and fruits so long as they have no chemical preservatives. Choose a colorful assortment because plants of different color provide you with various phytochemicals and varied benefits. Frozen fruits and veggie options are good too, but you should keep of canned foods. And dried fruits can cause weight gain because they are full of sugar.

Seeds and nuts make excellent choices for both snacks and additions to meals as they are great for your health. Legumes and foods made from them are fine too as long as it's made without chemicals or added sugar.

Also, you can eat grains on the whole foods diet. Though grains get a bad reputation, whole wheat, brown rice, oats, and barley in their natural form are good for you.

Try to keep of factory-farmed meats. As an alternative, settle for grass-fed meats that tend to be a little bit more costly. Still, you can spend the same amount of money by consuming less meat. The differences in taste and impact on your health are tremendous. Also, try to consume free-range or organic eggs.

Fish and seafood are valuable resources of protein and heart-healthy Omega 3 fatty acids. Most of them are considered lean protein, except oily fish. Shrimps are low in fat and calories but higher in cholesterol than lean meats.

While many people believe that milk, cheese, and yogurt are essential to maintaining bone health dairy apparently is in a grey zone. Almost all people are lactose intolerant to some degree. More often than not, removing lactose from your diet can cause a positive change of your state and energy level. Though, kefir, yogurt, and hard cheeses could be a decent alternative for the lactose intolerant by virtue of fermenting process.

Another problem with dairy is an allergic reaction to casein, one of the milk's proteins. And this can cause hormonal imbalance that can affect breast and prostate health. Contrary to this, it is believed that casein in goat milk has some different form, so it causes less or even no problems. In general, people who are intolerant to cow's dairy don't have any issues with the goat milk.

Junk food, by definition, is a processed food with low nutritional value. At the same time, these foods are high in calories, fat, sugar and salt.

Most packaged, or canned foods go through refining and processing with an eye to extend their shelf life. Moreover, manufacturers tend to add some deleterious substances in order to enhance the flavor of foods and increase profit.

For example, industrial trans-fat is used widely by many food fabricators. Trans fat or hydrogenated fat is a vegetable oil blasted with molecules of hydrogen. At all costs, avoid this artificial lipid, because they lead to heart disease and obesity. In fact, they are more harmful to our health than rich in cholesterol foods. And here is the tricky part: technically hydrogenated fats are not saturated, so on the food label they look like healthy fat. Besides, many low-fat foods are loaded with trans-fats and extra sugar. Unfortunately, this happens quite frequently with dairy products, frozen meals, crisps, margarine, sweets, cakes, biscuits and fried foods. Eating whole foods meals that are free from these detrimental trans-fats is a real benefit for your health.

Stay away from all foods from fast food restaurants such as McDonald's, Burger King, Taco Bell, Wendy's, and Arby's. Cooking your meals at home is the best way to ensure that you are consuming whole foods. Do not eat added sugar and artificial sweeteners.

Consider limiting your alcohol intake; entirely avoid consuming it for the first 30 days on the whole foods diet. Alcohol can cause damage to your digestive tract, liver, and heart. Inform your family and friends about your restriction so that they don't force you to drink. If you have a problem with drinking, consider visiting a therapist.

Sleep is often an underestimated aspect of life. Many people end up compromising on their night sleep and indulge in watching TV or communicating through social media. However, if you are thinking about whole foods diet benefits, you should plan an earlier bedtime too. Sufficient sleep increases the healing capacity of your body. Your metabolism and rest are controlled by the same centers of your brain. That's why the lack of sleep leads to weight gain. Try to sleep better, and you can certainly live better.

Water is the most essential substance in your body, so you have to remain hydrated as possible to maintain optimal cell health. There is no substitute for water, so you have to drink water all the time. Make sure that you drink 8 to 10 glasses of water daily and remain well hydrated. Drinking that amount allows your liver to break down fats more efficiently. Most likely you will need additional water in order to compensate for heat and caffeinated beverages.

Workouts help with increasing muscle function and reducing the fat content in your body. You can choose exercises and physical training program you wish to follow; the aim here is to provide enough physical activity on a daily basis in order to improve and maintain a healthy body.

It's crucial to supplement your whole foods diet with physical activity on a daily basis. Many people fail to get any physical activity but doing so is probably one of the worst things you can do to your body. Did you know that sedentary lifestyle is responsible for even more annual deaths than smoking? All types of physical training could be divided into three categories: cardio, strength, and flexibility.

Cardio workout is one of the most effective ways to burn away body fat. Usually, day-to-day cardio exercises are associated with running on a treadmill or elliptical. However, in reality, there are lots of other types of cardio activities; some of them you can do without specialized equipment or even without leaving your house. These exercises are designed to get your heart rate up and force our bodies to melt away the fat.

Dancing is fun and extremely effective cardio exercise. You can join a dance class or just use dance workout DVD at home. In the context of exercise, it actually doesn't matter what genre of dance you choose. Street dance, tango, or belly dancing – all are good. Anyway, as you move your body while dancing, you train your muscles, burn fat, and improve your balance and coordination.

Swimming is one of the best aerobic exercises; it provides you with all benefits of a cardio workout. At the same time, swimming reduces the impact on your joints due to relatively weightlessness. So it's an ideal exercise for those who experience joint pains during regular workouts such as knee pain while running. You even may not realize that hard work you are doing in a swimming pool. Still, you shouldn't exert too much effort on the first workouts. Instead work your way up gradually.

Playing sports can help you lose excess weight and also get rid of stress. It can be any type of playing sports of your choice including tennis or basketball. In fact, while playing your favorite game, you can benefit not just physically, but emotionally too. Train with your friends, family or find a partner to join in with you.

Remember that you have to warm up before taking up cardio or strengthen workouts. Know your limits and stop before you feel too tired. Take your time and you will get all positive benefits.

Weight training is associated with strength and muscular body. Obviously, weightlifting is more efficient for building muscles than cardio exercise. When we get older, we start losing muscle mass. So, it's a good idea to lift weights in order to tone muscles and strengthen. Always start with weights that you are comfortable lifting. If you are taking it up for the first time, it's important for you to work closely with a trainer.

Pilates does an excellent job in improving joint mobility and muscle elasticity. Slow light movements are not too imposing; you actually learn how to control these movements. Also, Pilates develops strong core and back muscles. As a result, you will get flat midsection and improved posture; it even eases back pain.

Did you know that famous McDonald's French fries have about twenty ingredients? When we prepare our food, we are in control of components going into our food. Naturally, if you cook at home, you will eat much healthier meals.

Eating together creates a healthy psychological climate in your family; everybody has time to talk about his or her day. Involve your kids in food preparation in order to teach them healthy eating habits.

Besides that, homemade foods are usually much cheaper than processed foods from a store and restaurant meals. It's really not necessary for you to pay the costs of running foods companies business.

For busy people, the most significant benefit of using Instant Pot is probably time-saving. Indeed, you can prepare a slow-cooker recipe that usually takes five or six hours just in one hour. This fantastic appliance has operation buttons for all most common cooking tasks. Also, Instant Pot allows you to plan your meals ahead by delayed cooking option. That means you don't even have to stand around in the kitchen to make your meal.

Another substantial benefit is that Instant Pot retains vitamins, minerals, and phytochemicals in your meals; even cooked greens retain their bright colors. Like with nutrients, the original juice and aroma of ingredients remain within your foods due to the cooking in a fully sealed environment.

Besides, steaming softens the foods, so the meat and even bones could be prepared really tender. Whole grains and beans also get soft texture easily.

Instant Pot is a high energy-efficient appliance, and it works quietly. You can save your money on electricity and also save on purchasing other kitchen appliance just by using this multi-cooker. Eventually, you have more chances to keep your kitchen clean and well-organized with Instant Pot.

When using your Instant Pot for pressure cooking, never fill the pot more than a 2/3rds. The reason to do so is that your Instant Pot needs some headspace to build pressure. Also, this is a safety feature; you can see a certain max fill line inside the pot.

Many recipes from this book say "cook on high pressure for..." In these cases, press the "Manual" or "Pressure Cook" button. Then press the plus or minus buttons in order to adjust the cooking time. In ten seconds the cooker will beep and start cooking.

When your Instant Pot finished preparing food, it switches to "Keep Warm" mode. This mode doesn't slow down natural pressure release. If you need to change something, just hit "Cancel."

Add soup to the beginning of your meal; this may help you consume fewer calories than usual. People who eat soup regularly less tend to be overweight than people who avoid soup. The combination of water and solids in soup increases a portion size without increasing calorie content. Also, soup fills you up more efficiently and for longer than regular solid foods. That's why soup makes up a substantial part of many weight loss diets.

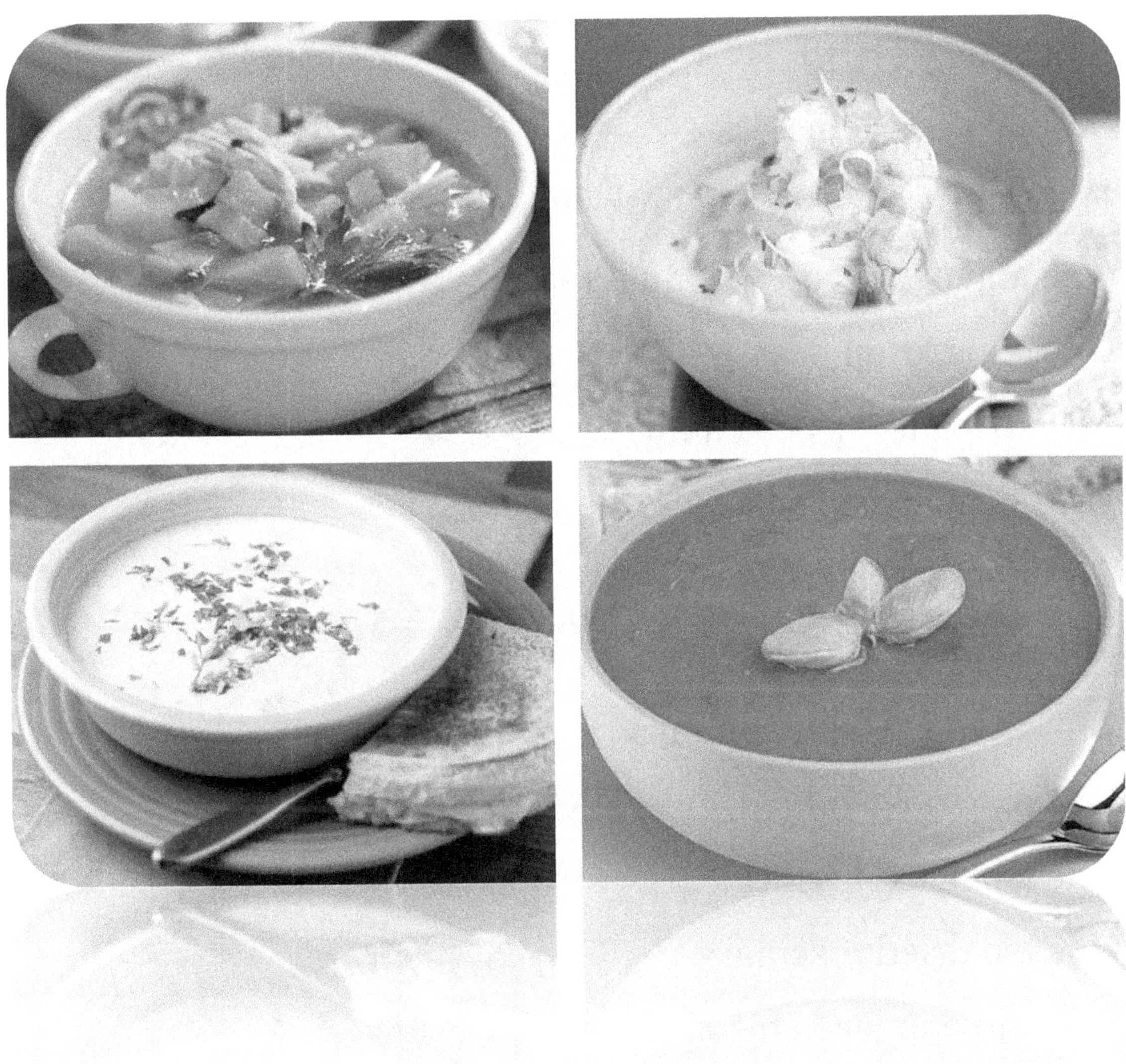

Chicken Soup with Veggies and Mushrooms

Time: 40 mins

Number of servings: 4

Ingredients:

One and a half pound cubed boneless and skinless chicken thighs

Six cups chicken stock

Four cups sliced cremini mushrooms

One and a half cup coconut cream

One cup frozen peas

Five tbsp all-purpose flour

Four diced carrots

Three stalks chopped celery

Three cloves minced garlic

One chopped white onion

One tbsp olive oil

One tsp dried thyme

One tsp dried rosemary

Salt and pepper to taste

Directions:

- Set your Instant Pot to sauté then add olive oil.

- When the oil gets hot, add veggies and sauté for five minutes without closing the lid. Then throw in garlic.

- Toss chicken in some flour. Add chicken, stock, thyme, and rosemary and stir well.

- Turn off sauté mode and close the lid. Set on manual and cook on high pressure for fifteen minutes. Whisk flour with one cup of broth.

- Allow to release pressure naturally and then open a lid. Set to sauté on medium and stir the mixture into the pot. Then add coconut cream and frozen peas.

- Let it simmer until thickened. Serve hot and enjoy!

Time: 30 mins

Number of servings: 6

Ingredients:

Four whole sun-dried tomatoes (not oil-packed!)

Two 15-oz cans of diced tomatoes with all juice

Two and a half cups vegetable stock

One chopped onion

One chopped rib celery

One chopped carrot

Two and a half tbsp butter

Two tbsp all-purpose flour

One tsp dried basil

Half tsp dried marjoram

Half tsp freshly ground pepper

Pinch of baking soda

Salt to taste

Directions:

• Sauté onion in your Instant Pot for two minutes. Then add celery, carrots, basil, and marjoram. Now sauté for four minutes.

- Then add the flour in and cook for one minute. Then add the rest of the ingredients.

- Select manual mode to cook on high pressure for eight minutes.

- Make a natural release of pressure. Then blend your soup until smooth in the food processor.

- Serve and enjoy!

Time: 20 mins

Number of servings: 4

Ingredients:

Three chopped beets

One cup red lentils

Six cups vegetable stock

Two chopped carrots

One chopped red onion

Three tbsp dark miso

One and a half tbsp chopped parsley

One tbsp sesame oil

Half tsp chopped thyme leaves

Three bay leaves

Salt and pepper to taste

Directions:

•   Add oil in your Instant Pot and set on sauté mode. Add onion and cook for five minutes.

•   Now add beets, carrots, stock, lentils, thyme, bay leaves, salt, and pepper. Stir well, close the lid and cook on high pressure for five minutes.

- Allow to release pressure naturally and then open a lid. Remove bay leaf from the pot and puree the soup using an immersion blender. Add miso mixed with some water and parsley, stir well.

- Serve and enjoy!

Time: 25 mins

Number of servings: 4

Ingredients:

Six big sliced mushrooms

One cup chopped tomatoes

Two chopped carrots

Two chopped celery sticks

One chopped brown onion

One cup chopped kale leaves

Four minced garlic cloves

Four cups veggie stock

One chopped zucchini

One half of red chili, chopped

A handful dried porcini mushrooms

A handful chopped parsley

One tbsp coconut oil

One tsp lemon zest

One bay leaf

Salt and pepper to taste

Directions:

- Add oil into your Instant Pot and select sauté mode to heat it up.

- Add carrots, celery, onion, and salt with pepper. Stir and cook for one minute. Then add all mushrooms, chili, garlic and cook for two minutes.

- Now add stock, tomatoes, zucchini, kale leaves, and bay leaf. Stir well, close the lid and cook at High for ten minutes.

- Allow to release pressure naturally and then open a lid. Add lemon zest and serve with parsley on top.

Lentil Soup without Meat

Time: 20 mins

Number of servings: 4

Ingredients:

One cup frozen corn

One cup red lentils

One cup brown lentils

Two chopped carrots

One cubed potato

One chopped medium onion

Six cups vegetable stock

Two tbsp olive oil

One bay leaf

Pinch of thyme

Salt and pepper to taste

Directions:

•   Pour olive oil in your Instant Pot and select sauté mode. Add carrots and sauté for two minutes.

•   Now add stock, all lentils, potato, thyme, and bay leaf. Stir well, close the lid and select Soup function. Cook for six minutes.

- Allow to release pressure naturally and open the lid. Remove bay leaf from the soup, add corn and salt with pepper.

- Stir well, serve, and enjoy!

Time: 30 mins

Number of servings: 4

Ingredients:

Five washed and trimmed artichoke hearts

One cup chopped gold potatoes

Half cup chopped shallots

One sliced leek

Six minced garlic cloves

Five tbsp butter

Quarter cup of cream

Twelve cups chicken stock

Four parsley springs

Two thyme springs

One bay leaf

Salt and pepper to taste

Directions:

• Set your Instant Pot on sauté mode, add butter and melt it.

• Add artichoke hearts, garlic, leek, and shallots. Stir well and brown for four minutes.

- Now add stock, potatoes, thyme, bay leaf, parsley, and salt with pepper. Stir again and cook on high for fifteen minutes.

- Release the pressure, gently open the lid and discard the bay leaf. Then blend your soup using an immersion blender.

- Finally, add cream, stir well, serve and enjoy!

Time: 40 mins

Number of servings: 4

Ingredients:

One pound ground pastured pork

Half head cabbage, chopped

Two cups shredded carrots

One diced onion

Four cups chicken broth

Half cup coconut aminos

One tbsp olive oil

One tsp onion powder

One tsp garlic powder

One tsp ground ginger

Directions:

• Pour olive oil in your Instant Pot. Select sauté mode and brown ground pork with onion until meat is no longer pink.

• Now add the rest of ingredients and stir well. Close the lid and cook at High pressure for twenty-five minutes.

• Use quick release the pressure, serve, and enjoy!

Time: 40 mins

Number of servings: 6

Ingredients:

One pound shelled and cut into 1-inch pieces shrimps

One 15-oz can crushed tomatoes

One cup coconut milk

Half cup long-grain rice

One chopped onion

One chopped bell pepper

Juice of one lemon

Four minced garlic cloves

Four cups water

Half cup chopped fresh parsley

Two tbsp olive oil

Two tsp salt

A pinch of ground black pepper

A pinch of red pepper flakes

Directions:

•   Heat the olive oil in your Instant Pot. Select sauté mode and add bell pepper, onion, and garlic. Cook until the pepper and onion are soft.

•   Now add water, tomatoes, rice, red pepper flakes, and salt to the pot and bring to a boil. Then cook on high for 10 minutes.

•   Stir the coconut milk into the soup. Bring to a simmer again and then stir in the shrimp. Simmer for five minutes stirring occasionally.

•   Stir in the juice of one lemon, parsley, and black pepper. Serve and enjoy!

Time: 30 mins

Number of servings: 6

Ingredients:

One pound soaked overnight dried black beans

Five chopped tomatoes

One chopped red onion

One chopped red bell pepper

Five minced garlic cloves

Four cups water

Half cup red wine

Two tbsp sherry vinegar

Two tbsp olive oil

One bay leaf

Two tsp dried oregano

One tsp ground cumin

Salt and pepper to taste

Directions:

• Heat the oil in your Instant Pot. Add red bell pepper, onion, garlic, bay leaf, oregano, cumin and sauté for five minutes.

•   Now add water, beans, wine, vinegar, salt, and pepper. Close the pot lid and cook at High pressure for fifteen minutes.

•   Allow to release pressure naturally and then open a lid. Use an immersion blender to crush the black beans in your soup partially.

•   Serve with tomatoes and enjoy!

Time: 40 mins

Number of servings: 8

Ingredients:

Half pound diced crimini mushrooms

Half cup pearl barley

One diced onion

One diced celery stalk

One diced carrot

Three minced garlic cloves

Four cups chicken stock

Two thyme sprigs

One sage sprig

Salt and pepper to taste

Directions:

•   Put all ingredients in your Instant Pot. Select manual mode and cook on high pressure for twenty minutes.

•   Allow to release pressure naturally and then open a lid. Stir well, serve, and enjoy!

Time: 30 mins

Number of servings: 6

Ingredients:

One and a half pounds ground chicken breast

Two whisked eggs

Two chopped yellow onions

Three chopped carrots

Four chopped celery stalks

One bunch kale, chopped

Two minced garlic cloves

Six cups chicken stock

Two tbsp nutritional yeast

Two tbsp olive oil

Two tbsp arrowroot powder

Half tbsp dried basil

Half tbsp dried oregano

Two tsp dried thyme

One tsp garlic powder

One tsp onion powder

One tsp crushed red pepper

Salt and black pepper to taste

Directions:

• Set your Instant Pot on sauté mode, add olive oil and heat it up. Then add carrots, celery, onions, stir and cook for three minutes.

• Now add stock, kale, garlic, half tsp red pepper, and salt with black pepper. Stir well and continue cooking.

• In a bowl mix ground meat with arrow powder, garlic powder, onion powder, oregano, basil, yeast, half tsp red pepper, salt, black pepper and stir well. Shape meatballs with your hands and gently drop them into the soup.

• Close the pot lid and cook on High for fifteen minutes. Then release pressure, open the lid and set it on sauté again.

• Add eggs, stir and cook for two minutes.

• Serve hot and enjoy!

Time: 30 mins

Number of servings: 2

Ingredients:

Seven chopped celery stalks

Three chopped potatoes

One chopped yellow onion

Four cups vegetable stock

One tbsp olive oil

One tsp curry powder

One tsp celery seeds

A handful of chopped parsley

Salt and pepper to taste

Directions:

• Add oil in your Instant Pot and select sauté mode.

• Add celery seeds, onion, and curry powder. Stir and cook for one minute.

• Now add potatoes and celery stalks. Stir and cook for five minutes.

• Add stock, salt, and pepper. Close the pot lid and cook on High for ten minutes.

- Release the pressure, open the lid and blend your soup with an immersion blender.

- Add parsley, stir, serve, and enjoy!

Time: 50 mins

Number of servings: 6

Ingredients:

Three 15-oz cans drained navy beans

Three cups baby spinach

Four slices center cut bacon, chopped

One chopped onion

One chopped carrot

One chopped celery stalk

Four cups chicken stock

Two tbsp tomato paste

Two bay leaves

One fresh rosemary sprig

Directions:

- In a blender, blend one can of beans with one can water.

- In your Instant Pot sauté the bacon until crisp. Then transfer it to a plate.

- Add carrot, onion, celery and sauté for five minutes.

- Then add stock, pureed and remaining beans, tomato paste, bay leaves, and rosemary. Close the pot lid and cook on high pressure for fifteen minutes.

- Allow the pressure to release naturally and open the lid. Remove rosemary and bay leaves. Blend two cups of the soup in your blender and then put them back to the pot.

- Add spinach, serve topped with bacon and enjoy!

Time: 35 mins

Number of servings: 3

Ingredients:

Eight cups thinly sliced yellow onions

Six cups pork stock

Two tbsp coconut oil

One tbsp balsamic vinegar

One tsp salt

Two bay leaves

Two large sprigs of fresh thyme

Directions:

• Add coconut oil in your Instant Pot and select sauté mode.

• Add onions and sauté for fifteen minutes, stirring once in a while, until transparent.

• Scrape up browned-up onions. Add balsamic vinegar, stock, salt, thyme and bay leaves.

• Close the pot lid and cook on High for ten minutes. Then allow the pressure to release naturally and open the lid.

• Remove thyme stems and bay leaves. Blend the soup until smooth and serve.

Time: 30 mins

Number of servings: 4

Ingredients:

One pound chopped carrots

One chopped onion

One minced garlic clove

Two cups chicken stock

One small ginger piece, grated

One 14-oz can of coconut milk

One tbsp olive oil

One tbsp butter

One tbsp Sriracha sauce

A handful of chopped cilantro leaves

A pinch of brown sugar

Salt and pepper to taste

Directions:

- Add butter and olive oil in your Instant Pot and select sauté mode. Add onion, stir and cook for three minutes.

- Add garlic and ginger, then stir and cook for one minute.

- Now add carrots, sugar, salt, and pepper. Stir and cook for two minutes.

- Add coconut milk, stock, and sriracha sauce. Close the pot lid and cook on High for six minutes.

- Allow the pressure to release naturally and open the lid. Blend your soup with an immersion blender. Serve topped with cilantro and enjoy!

Time: 40 mins

Number of servings: 4

Ingredients:

One pound chopped beef stew meat

Three cups mixed carrots, onion and celery

Ten diced baby bell mushrooms

Eight minced garlic cloves

One chopped potato

Half cup barley

Six cup beef stock

Two tbsp olive oil

Two bay leaves

Half tsp dried thyme

Salt and pepper to taste

Directions:

• Add oil in your Instant Pot and select sauté mode. Add meat, salt, and pepper. Stir well, cook for three minutes then transfer to a plate.

• Add mushrooms, brown them for two minutes and transfer to a plate too.

•   Add mixed carrots, onion, and celery to the pot and cook for four minutes. Then put back to the pot meat and mushrooms and stir everything.

•   Now add stock, potatoes, barley, bay leaves, thyme, salt, and pepper. Stir well, close the pot lid and cook on High for twenty minutes.

•   Allow the pressure to release naturally and open the lid. Stir the soup, serve and enjoy!

Time: 30 mins

Number of servings: 6

Ingredients:

Six ears fresh corn

Two diced potatoes

Four cooked and diced slices bacon

Half cup chopped onion

Three cups water

Three cups milk

Four tbsp butter

Two tbsp cornstarch

Two tbsp fresh parsley

Salt and pepper to taste

Directions:

• Shuck the corn and take a sharp knife to cut off the kernels.

• Add the butter in your Instant Pot and select sauté mode. Add the chopped onions and cook for three minutes, stirring occasionally.

• Now add three cups water and corncobs. Close the pot lid and cook on High for ten minutes. Then do a quick pressure release and open the lid. Carefully remove corncobs from the pot.

• Add potatoes and corn kernels. Close the pot lid and cook on High for four minutes. Meanwhile, in a small bowl, mix together cornstarch and two tbsp water.

• Do a quick pressure release and select simmer mode. Stir in cornstarch mixture, milk, bacon, and parsley. Add salt and pepper, serve, and enjoy!

Time: 30 mins

Number of servings: 6

Ingredients:

One pound ground beef

Half pound ground pork

One medium cabbage, chopped

Two 15-oz cans diced fire roasted tomatoes, not drained

Two cups cauliflower crumbles

One chopped onion

Three minced cloves garlic

Four cups beef stock

Three tbsp tomato paste

One tbsp olive oil

Two tsp onion powder

Two tsp garlic powder

One tsp oregano

One tsp thyme

Half tsp cayenne pepper

One bay leaf

Salt and pepper to taste

Directions:

•   Add olive oil in your Instant Pot and select sauté mode. Add beef and pork and cook until it brown. Add garlic powder, onion powder, thyme, oregano, cayenne pepper, bay leaf, garlic to the meat.

•   Add stock, cabbage, onion, cauliflower crumbles, tomatoes and tomato paste. Close the pot lid and cook on High for fifteen minutes.

•   Allow the pressure to release naturally and open the lid. Serve hot and enjoy!

Time: 35 mins

Number of servings: 4

Ingredients:

16-oz fresh halibut, cut into thick chunks

Two cups shredded carrots

Two finely chopped stalks celery

One chopped zucchini

One chopped onion

One chopped red bell pepper

One 15-oz can of diced tomatoes, not drained

Six cups chicken stock

Two tbsp olive oil

Two tsp Cajun seasoning

A handful of fresh parsley

Salt and pepper to taste

Directions:

• Add olive oil in your Instant Pot and select sauté mode. Add onion, carrots, celery and cook for five minutes, stirring occasionally.

•   Add red pepper and cook five minutes more. Then add stock, tomatoes, zucchini, seasonings. Bring to a boil, cover and simmer for five minutes.

•   Add fish and close the lid. Cook for ten minutes. Garnish with parsley, serve, and enjoy!

Time: 60 mins

Number of servings: 4

Ingredients:

Two pounds chopped in half asparagus

One diced white onion

Five pressed cloves garlic

One cup diced ham

Four cups chicken stock

Three tbsp ghee

Half tsp dried thyme

Salt and pepper to taste

Directions:

• Add ghee in your Instant Pot and select sauté mode. Add onion and cook it for five minutes.

• Add stock, ham. And garlic. Simmer for three minutes. Then add asparagus along with the thyme.

• Close the pot lid and cook on Soup setting for forty-five minutes. Do a quick pressure release, open the lid and stir everything until smooth.

• Serve and enjoy!

Some people don't follow a vegetarian diet permanently, but occasionally they are just looking to go meatless. Naturally, vegetarian diet contains more fiber, healthy micronutrients, and antioxidants from plant-based foods. Some of these recipes include cheese or butter, which are not allowed for a vegan diet. At the same time, lacto-ovo vegetarians are allowed to consume eggs and dairy. Surely, you can use these recipes as side dishes for your meat, fish, and poultry.

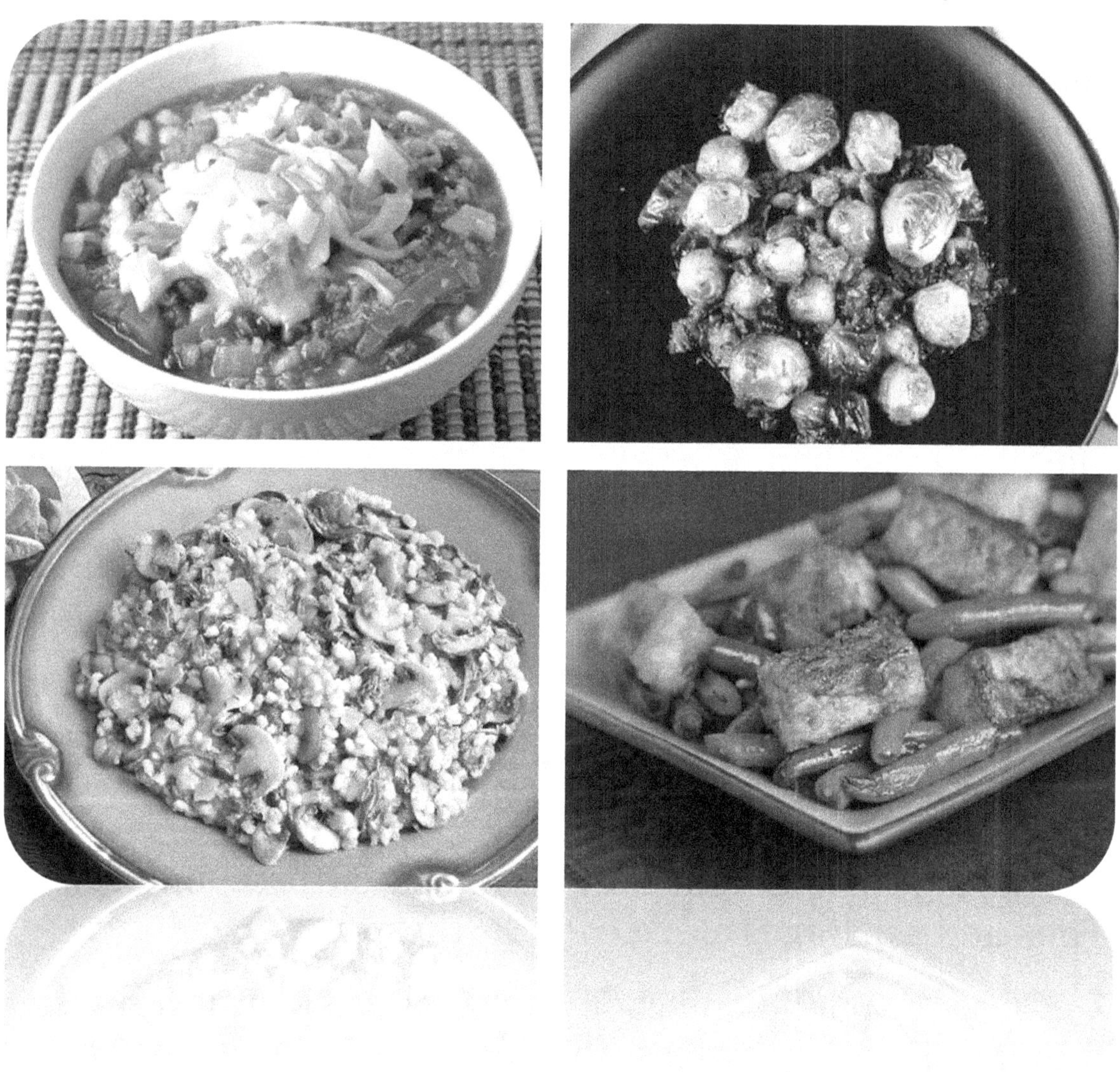

Time: 40 mins

Number of servings: 4

Ingredients:

One cup pearl barley

Two cups chopped yellow onions

Two tbsp black barley

Quarter cup grated parmesan

One 1.5-oz pack dried mushrooms

Two cups dry sherry

Two cups water

One tbsp olive oil

One tsp fennel seeds

Salt and pepper to taste

Directions:

• Add oil in your Instant Pot and select sauté mode. Add onions and fennel seeds, cook for four minutes.

• Add water, sherry, barley, black barley, mushrooms, salt, pepper, and stir well. Cover the lid and cook on high for eighteen minutes.

• Release the pressure and set pot on simmer mode. Cook for five more minutes.

- Serve topped with parmesan and enjoy!

Time: 10 mins

Number of servings: 4

Ingredients:

One pound Brussels sprouts

One tbsp olive oil

Four tbsp pine nuts

One cup of water

Salt and pepper to taste

Directions:

• Pour water into your Instant Pot and set the steamer basket. Then put Brussels sprouts in a steamer basket.

• Close the lid and select manual mode. Cook for three minutes. Then use rapid pressure release.

• Transfer Brussels sprouts to the plate. Add pine nuts, olive oil, salt, and pepper. Serve and enjoy!

Time: 40 mins

Number of servings: 4

Ingredients:

Six cups baby spinach

One cup rinsed brown lentils

Two chopped carrots

Four minced garlic cloves

One chopped celery stalk

One chopped yellow onion

Two tbsp olive oil

Four cups vegetable stock

Two tsp cumin

One tsp turmeric

One tsp thyme

Salt and pepper to taste

Directions:

• Add oil in your Instant Pot and select sauté mode. Add onion, carrots, and celery. Stir and cook for five minutes.

• Now add garlic, cumin, turmeric, thyme, salt, and pepper. Stir and cook for one minute more.

- Add lentils and stock. Close the pot lid and cook on High for twelve minutes.

- Allow the pressure to release naturally and open the lid. Add spinach, serve and enjoy!

Time: 25 mins

Number of servings: 4

Ingredients:

One pound green beans

One and a half cup sliced mushrooms

One chopped onion

Half cup pureed tofu

Two tbsp olive oil

One cup vegetable stock

Directions:

•   Add olive oil in your Instant Pot and select sauté mode. Add mushrooms and onions and cook for three minutes.

•   Now add stock, pureed tofu, and green beans. Stir well, close the lid, and cook on high for fifteen minutes.

•   Use rapid pressure release and open the lid. Mix well, serve and enjoy!

Time: 30 mins

Number of servings: 4

Ingredients:

One cup rinsed bulgur

Half cup chopped scallions

Half cup chopped almonds

Juice from two oranges

Zest from one orange

Two minced garlic cloves

Two tbsp grated ginger

Half cup water

Two tsp canola oil

One tbsp soy sauce

Salt to taste

Directions:

• Add oil in your Instant Pot and select sauté mode. Add garlic and ginger, stir and cook for one minute.

• Now add water, bulgur, and orange juice. Stir, close the pot lid and cook on High for five minutes.

- Meanwhile, heat up a pan and toast almonds for three minutes over medium heat. Then add scallions, orange zest, soy sauce and salt. Stir and cook for one minute.

- Allow the pressure to release naturally and open the lid of the pot. Add the mix from your pan to bulgur. Stir well with a fork, serve, and enjoy!

Time: 25 mins

Number of servings: 6

Ingredients:

One 15-oz can black beans

One can diced tomatoes

Half cup quinoa

Three peeled and chopped sweet potatoes

Two chopped celery stalks

One chopped onion

One chopped bell pepper

Two minced garlic cloves

Two tbsp tomato paste

Four cups vegetable stock

Two tsp ground cumin

Two tsp paprika

One tsp chili powder

One tsp ground coriander

Salt to taste

Directions:

- Put all the ingredients in your Instant Pot and stir well. Close the lid and cook at high pressure for twelve minutes.

- Use rapid pressure release and open the lid carefully. Stir well, serve, and enjoy!

Time: 20 mins

Number of servings: 4

Ingredients:

One cup rinsed coucous

Two chopped red onion

Two chopped red pepper

Two cups veggie stock

Two tbsp red wine vinegar

Half tsp sesame oil

Half tsp ground cinnamon

A pinch of ground coriander

Salt and pepper to taste

Directions:

• Add oil in your Instant Pot and select sauté mode. Add onion and bell pepper. Stir and cook for five minutes.

• Add stock, couscous, coriander, cinnamon, vinegar, salt, and pepper. Stir, close the lid and cook at high for three minutes.

• Allow the pressure to release in a natural way, and then open the pot lid. Serve and enjoy!

Time: 40 mins

Number of servings: 4

Ingredients:

One pound soaked overnight pinto beans

One can chopped tomatoes

One chopped onion

Two tbsp olive oil

Four cups water

Half tsp garlic powder

Half tsp oregano

Half tsp dried sage

Salt and pepper to taste

Directions:

•   Pour one tbsp oil in your Instant Pot and select sauté mode. Add onion and sauté for five minutes.

•   Add water, pinto beans, tomatoes, garlic powder, oregano sage, salt, pepper, and another tbsp olive oil. Close the lid and select bean/chili mode and cook at high pressure for thirty minutes.

•   Use rapid pressure release method. Serve warm and enjoy!

Time: 45 mins

Number of servings: 6

Ingredients:

One and a half cups wheat berries

One cup cut into halves cherry tomatoes

Half cup crumbled feta cheese

Half cup pitted and chopped kalamata olives

Two chopped green onions

Two tbsp olive oil

Four cups water

One tbsp balsamic vinegar

One handful chopped basil leaves

One handful chopped parsley

Salt and pepper to taste

Directions:

• Add one tbsp oil in your Instant Pot and select sauté mode. Add wheat berries, stir, and cook for five minutes.

• Now add water, salt, pepper. Close the pot lid and cook on High for thirty minutes.

- Allow the pressure to release naturally and open the lid of the pot. Put wheat berries in a salad bowl.

- Add one tbsp olive oil, tomatoes, balsamic vinegar, green onions, olives, cheese, parsley, basil, salt, and pepper. Toss to coat and serve right away!

Time: 45 mins

Number of servings: 4

Ingredients:

One cup rinsed chickpeas

Four minced garlic cloves

Four cups water

Two bay leaves

Salt to taste

Directions:

•   Put all ingredients into your Instant Pot. Close the lid and select bean/chili mode. Cook for thirty five minutes.

•   Allow the pressure to release naturally and open the lid of the pot. Serve chickpeas with steamed rice and enjoy!

Time: 15 mins

Number of servings: 4

Ingredients:

Two cups quinoa

Four cups chopped spinach

Half cup crumbled feta cheese

Half cup pitted and chopped black olives

Two chopped tomatoes

Three chopped celery stalks

One chopped red bell pepper

Half cup pesto

Two cups vegetable stock

A handful of sliced almonds

Salt to taste

Directions:

•   Put stock, quinoa, bell pepper, celery, salt and spinach in your Instant Pot. Close the lid and cook on high for two minutes.

•   Allow the pressure to release in a natural way and open the lid. Add tomatoes, pesto, stir well and transfer to plates.

- Now add cheese and toss to coat. Serve topped with almonds and enjoy!

Time: 20 mins

Number of servings: 4

Ingredients:

One pound cut into 2-inch pieces butternut squash

Two peeled and sliced apples

One sliced onion

Two tbsp coconut oil

One cup water

Pinch of cinnamon

Pinch of ginger

Directions:

•   Pour water into your Instant Pot and place a steamer basket. Put in the steamer basket butternut squash, apples, and onion.

•   Close the pot lid and cook on High for eight minutes. Then use rapid pressure release. Open the pot and transfer mixture to a bowl.

•   Now use a masher, add coconut oil, ginger, and cinnamon. Mix well, serve warm and enjoy!

Time: 30 mins

Number of servings: 4

Ingredients:

One cup hulled barley, rinsed

One cup spinach pesto

Three chopped celery stalks

One chopped green apple

Three cups water

Salt and white pepper to taste

Directions:

• Put barley, water, salt and pepper in your Instant Pot. Close the lid and cook on high for twenty minutes.

• Use rapid pressure release and open the lid. Strain and put barley in a bowl.

• Add apple, celery, spinach pesto. Toss to coat and serve right away.

Time: 20 mins

Number of servings: 4

Ingredients:

Six cups chopped red cabbage

One chopped onion

Three minced garlic cloves

Half cup applesauce

One tbsp olive oil

One cup water

One tbsp apple cider vinegar

Salt and pepper to taste

Directions:

• Pour olive oil in your Instant Pot and select sauté mode. Add garlic and onion and cook for two minutes.

• Now add all remaining ingredients and stir well. Close the lid and cook on high pressure for ten minutes.

• Use rapid pressure release, stir, serve and enjoy!

Time: 25 mins

Number of servings: 4

Ingredients:

One cup steel cut oats

One chopped Thai green chili

One chopped carrot

Half green bell pepper, chopped

One inch ginger, grated

Two tbsp canola oil

One and a half cups water

Two curry leaves

Half tsp urad dal

A pinch of mustard seeds

A pinch of asafetida powder

A pinch of turmeric powder

Salt to taste

Directions:

• Put oats in your Instant Pot. Add water, close the lid and cook on high for seven minutes.

- Meanwhile, heat up a pan with the oil. Add mustard seeds, green chili, bell pepper, urdal dal, turmeric, curry leaves, ginger, carrot, asafetida powder. Stir and cook over medium heat for five minutes.

- Release pressure from the pot and open the lid. Add oats to the pan, stir, serve and enjoy!

Time: 20 mins

Number of servings: 2

Ingredients:

Half middle-size pumpkin, pureed

One cup quick oats

Half cup almond milk

One and a half cup water

One tbsp brown sugar

One tsp pumpkin pie spice

Directions:

• Put all the ingredients in your Instant Pot and stir well. Close the lid and cook on high for three minutes.

• Allow the pressure to release in a natural way and open the lid. Stir well and serve warm.

Time: 40 mins

Number of servings: 6

Ingredients:

Three pounds cut in half Yukon gold potatoes

Two cups washed green beans

One cup white wine

Half cup chopped chives

Quarter cup fresh dill

Four tbsp olive oil

Two tbsp rice vinegar

One tbsp whole grain mustard

Salt and pepper to taste

Directions:

• Pour one cup of water and place steamer basket in your Instant Pot. Put potatoes in the steamer basket, close the lid and cook on high for eight minutes.

• Allow the pressure to release in a natural way and open the lid. Carefully remove potatoes with tongs.

• Now add green beans, close the lid and cook on high for one minute. Then use rapid pressure release and remove steamer basket to cool it out.

- In a small pan, pour wine and simmer for six minutes, until reduced by half. Whisk together reduced wine, oil, and vinegar.

- In a bowl, combine potatoes, green beans, wine mixture, and herbs. Stir gently until thoroughly mixed.

- Serve and enjoy!

Time: 30 mins

Number of servings: 4

Ingredients:

Two cups lentils

Two cups chopped tomatoes

One chopped yellow onion

One chopped celery stalk

One chopped green bell pepper

Two tbsp olive oil

Two cups water

One tsp curry powder

Salt and pepper to taste

Directions:

• Add olive oil in your Instant Pot and select sauté mode. Add onion, celery, tomatoes, and bell pepper. Stir and cook for four minutes.

• Add water, lentils, curry, salt, and pepper. Stir, close the pot lid and cook on high for fifteen minutes.

• Allow the pressure to release naturally and open the lid. Stir well, serve and enjoy!

Creamy & Light Mashed Sweet Potatoes

Time: 40 mins

Number of servings: 2

Ingredients:

Five sweet potatoes, cut into big chunks

One 14-oz can coconut milk

Three tbsp coconut oil

One cup water

One tbsp cinnamon

One tsp ginger

Half tsp nutmeg

Salt to taste

Directions:

• Put sweet potatoes into your Instant Pot. Add water, coconut milk, oil, cinnamon, nutmeg, ginger, and salt.

• Close the lid and cook on high for twenty minutes. Then allow the pressure to release naturally and open the lid. Remove potatoes into a large bowl.

• Mash potatoes until desired consistency. Stir well, serve and enjoy!

Time: 20 mins

Number of servings: 4

Ingredients:

One cup lentils

One chopped red bell pepper

One chopped red onion

Three chopped celery stalks

Three minced garlic cloves

Two cups vegetable stock

Juice of one lemon

Two tbsp olive oil

Two tbsp chopped parsley

Half tsp dried oregano

Half tsp dried thyme

One bay leaf

Salt and pepper to taste

Directions:

• Put lentils, thyme and bay leaf in your Instant Pot. Pour stock, stir, close the lid and cook on high for eight minutes.

- Use rapid pressure release and open the lid. Drain lentils and put them in a large bowl.

- Add lemon juice, olive oil, onion, bell pepper, celery, garlic, parsley, oregano, salt, and pepper. Toss to coat, serve and enjoy!

Time: 30 mins

Number of servings: 4

Ingredients:

One small cauliflower, chopped into large florets

Two cubed potatoes

Two tomatoes

Half an onion, chopped

Six garlic cloves

Half of hot green chili

One inch ginger

One tsp olive oil

One tsp ground cumin

One tsp garam masala

Half tsp paprika

Half tsp turmeric

Salt to taste

Directions:

• Blend the tomatoes, onion, green chili, garlic, and ginger until smooth.

- Add oil in your Instant Pot and select sauté mode. Add the mixture from the blender, potato, and spices. Stir well and cook for five minutes.

- Add cauliflower and mix well. Close the pot lid and cook on high for two minutes. Then use rapid pressure release and open the lid.

- Serve hot with rice and enjoy!

Time: 10 mins

Number of servings: 2

Ingredients:

One pound new potatoes

Three tbsp coconut butter

One cup water

Three tsp garlic puree

Handful fresh herbs

Salt and pepper to taste

Directions:

•   Pour water in your Instant Pot and insert a steaming basket. Then put potatoes into steaming basket.

•   Add coconut butter, garlic puree, fresh herbs, salt, and pepper. Mix well everything.

•   Close the lid and cook on high for four minutes. Then allow the pressure to release naturally and open the lid. Serve garnished with fresh herbs and enjoy!

Time: 10 mins

Number of servings: 2

Ingredients:

Two cubed sweet potatoes

Two diced carrots

Six cups chopped kale

Four tbsp peanut butter

Four minced garlic cloves

Five cups vegetable stock

Two tbsp olive oil

Two tbsp honey

One tsp clove

One tsp ginger

One tsp cumin

Salt and pepper to taste

Directions:

• Add olive oil in your Instant Pot and select sauté mode. Add ginger and garlic, cook for one minute stirring constantly.

•   Now add cumin, clove, salt, and pepper. Continue cooking until spices are fragrant.

•   Add all the remaining ingredients, close the pot lid and cook on high for five minutes.

•   Allow the pressure to release in a natural way and open the lid. Serve and enjoy!

Creamy Mushroom Risotto

Time: 30 mins

Number of servings: 4

Ingredients:

One and a half pounds sliced mushrooms

Two cups Arobio rice

One chopped onion

One cup grated parmesan cheese

One tbsp butter

Two tbsp olive oil

Four cups vegetable stock

Quarter cup white wine

Two springs fresh thyme

Salt and pepper to taste

Directions:

• Add olive oil in your Instant Pot and select sauté mode. Add mushrooms and onion, stir and cook until the mushrooms have softened.

• Now add rice, salt, and pepper. Pour in the stock and the wine. Close the pot lid and cook on high pressure for seven minutes.

- Allow the pressure to release naturally and open the lid. Add cheese, butter, and seasoning. Serve and enjoy!

Time: 15 mins

Number of servings: 4

Ingredients:

One and a half cups Arborio rice

One cup broccoli florets

One cup sliced fresh peas

One cup diced leek

One cup spinach

One chopped onion

Two minced garlic cloves

One bunch asparagus, sliced

Half bunch chives, sliced

Four cups vegetable stock

Two tbsp olive oil

Four tbsp butter

Two tbsp lemon juice

One tsp lemon zest

One tsp fresh thyme

Half tsp garlic powder

A pinch of red pepper flakes

Directions:

- Pre-heat your oven to 400 °F. Then line a baking sheet with parchment paper. Place asparagus, peas, and broccoli on the baking sheet. Add one tsp olive oil, salt, pepper flakes and toss to coat. Place in the oven for twenty minutes then remove and set aside.

- Add remaining olive oil in your Instant Pot and select sauté. Add onions, garlic, leeks and cook for three minutes.

- Now add rice, stock, butter, and thyme. Stir well, close the pot lid and cook on high for seven minutes.

- Use quick pressure release and open the lid and stir well. Add roasted veggies, spinach, chives and spices to the rice. Cook, stirring often, for two minutes. Serve topped with lemon zest and enjoy!

Time: 25 mins

Number of servings: 4

Ingredients:

One cup Arborio rice

Two cups milk

Half cup honey

Two eggs

One cup water

One tbsp butter

One tsp vanilla extract

One tsp cinnamon

A handful of fresh berries or raisins

A pinch of salt

Directions:

• Add the butter in your Instant Pot and select sauté. Add rice and cook, stirring often, until toasted.

• Pour in one cup of milk and one cup of water. Add honey, salt, and spices. Close the pot lid and cook on high for fifteen minutes.

- In a bowl, whisk eggs with the remaining milk. Then strain the egg-milk mixture through a fine mesh strainer and set aside.

- Use rapid pressure release and open the lid. Select sauté again. Then whisk in the mix of egg and milk. Bring to a boil and simmer for one minute.

- Serve hot or cold. Top with raisins or fresh berries.

Time: 35 mins

Number of servings: 4

Ingredients:

Two cups brown long-grain rice

Half cup tomato paste

Half white onion, chopped

Three minced cloves garlic

One small jalapeño

Two cups water

Two tbsp olive oil

Two tsp salt

Directions:

• Add olive oil in your Instant Pot and select sauté. Add rice, onion, garlic, salt and cook for four minutes.

• Meanwhile, mix tomato paste and water until combined. Then pour into the pot. Add the whole jalapeño. Close the pot lid and cook on High for twenty-two minutes.

• Allow the pressure to release naturally and open the lid. Fluff rice with a fork, serve hot and enjoy!

Time: 75 mins

Number of servings: 6

Ingredients:

Two pounds peeled and chopped white potatoes

Two cups frozen peas, rinsed under warm water

Half cup tomato paste

Half cup chopped parsley

Six minced cloves garlic

Two chopped white onions

Three chopped carrots

Three ribs celery, chopped

Two sliced portabella mushrooms

Five cups water

Two tbsp olive oil

One tbsp paprika

One tbsp dried Italian herbs seasoning

Two tsp finely chopped fresh rosemary

Directions:

- Add olive oil in your Instant Pot and select sauté. Add celery, carrots, onions, and cook, stirring often, for three minutes. Then stir in the mushrooms and garlic and cook for five minutes.

- Add potatoes, water, tomato paste, Italian herbs, rosemary, and paprika. Close the pot lid and cook on High for twenty-five minutes.

- Allow the pressure to release naturally and open the lid. Add the peas and select the sauté mode again. Cook for five minutes.

- Blend two cups of your stew in a blender. Then stir the mixture back to the pot.

- Stir in the parsley, serve and enjoy!

Time: 25 mins

Number of servings: 6

Ingredients:

Two cups split peas, rinsed well

Half cup chopped tinned tomatoes

One chopped white onion

One cubed carrot

One chopped celery stalk

Five minced cloves garlic

Juice of half lemon

A bunch of scallions, chopped

Two tbsp olive oil

Seven cups vegetable stock

One and a half tsp cumin powder

One tsp paprika powder

One bay leaf

A pinch of cinnamon powder

A pinch of cayenne pepper

Salt to taste

Directions:

• Add olive oil in your Instant Pot and select sauté mode. Then add onion, carrot, celery, and cook, stirring occasionally, for four minutes.

• Now add the rest of ingredients, except scallions and stir well. Close the lid and cook on high for ten minutes.

• Allow the pressure to release in a natural way and open the lid. Serve with chopped scallions and enjoy!

Egg Recipes

Eggs are known to be one of the most nutritious foods on our planet. A whole egg contains more than 100 mg of Choline. This nutrient aids in building cell membranes and brain development, along with various other features. Your body produces very small amounts of Choline, and you need to get it from your food. Researches show that most people in the US get less than the recommended amount of Choline.

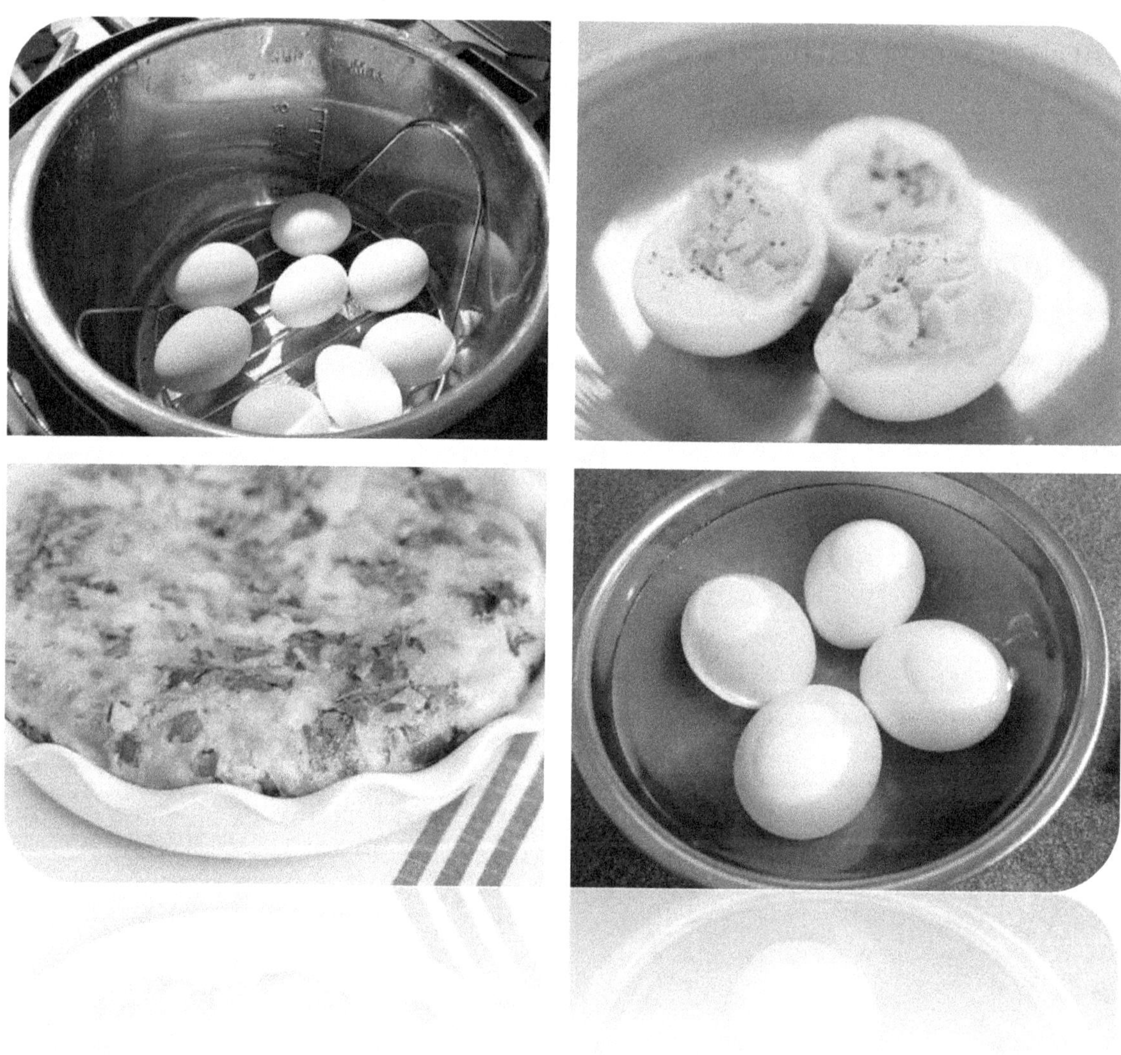

Time: 16 mins

Number of servings: 12

Ingredients:

Twelve eggs

One cup water

Directions:

• Add water in your Instant Pot. Place steam rack in the pot and put eggs on the rack. Close the lid and cook on high for six minutes.

• Allow the pressure to release naturally for five minutes then use rapid pressure release.

• Transfer eggs to a bowl filled with cold water for two minutes. Now you can peel boiled eggs easily.

Time: 25 mins

Number of servings: 24

Ingredients:

Twelve eggs

One cup water

Quarter cup sour cream

Two tbsp lime juice

Two tbsp melted butter

Two tbsp minced cilantro

One tbsp Dijon mustard

Salt to taste

Directions:

• Prepare hard-cooked eggs as described in the previous recipe. Peel eggs and slice in half lengthwise.

• In a bowl, mix together sour cream, Dijon mustard, melted butter, lime juice, cilantro, and salt. Stir well.

• Remove yolks and add them to the mixture in a bowl. Mash using a fork and stir until fully combined.

• Take a spoon to fill the egg whites with the yolk mixture. Serve immediately and enjoy!

Time: 20 mins

Number of servings: 4

Ingredients:

Six eggs

Six chopped slices bacon

Four chopped mushrooms

Half cup chopped parsley

Two cups frozen hash browns

Half cup shredded cheddar cheese

One and a half cup water

Quarter cup milk

One tbsp butter

Salt and pepper to taste

Directions:

• Add bacon in your Instant Pot and cook until crispy. Then add mushrooms and cook for three minutes. Now add hash browns and cook, stirring occasionally, for two minutes.

• In a bowl, whisk together eggs and milk. Then add bacon with veggies and mushrooms from the pot and stir well. Now add cheese, salt, and pepper.

- Grease a heatproof container with butter. Then pour in egg mixture.

- Pour water in your Instant Pot and set trivet inside. Place the heatproof container on the top of the trivet. Close the pot lid and cook on High for ten minutes.

- Use rapid pressure release and carefully remove the heatproof container. Dump out onto a large platter, serve topped with chopped parsley and enjoy!

Poultry is rich in highly digestible protein, Thiamin, vitamin B6, Pantothenic acid, zinc, iron, and cooper. Saturated fat mainly found in the skin and could be removed easily. So, if you are looking for a source of lean protein, the bird is the word. However, duck contains the higher amount of saturated fat than chicken. Also, chicken has been known to be a favorite protein source for many athletes and fitness practitioners; it's a most common type of poultry in the world.

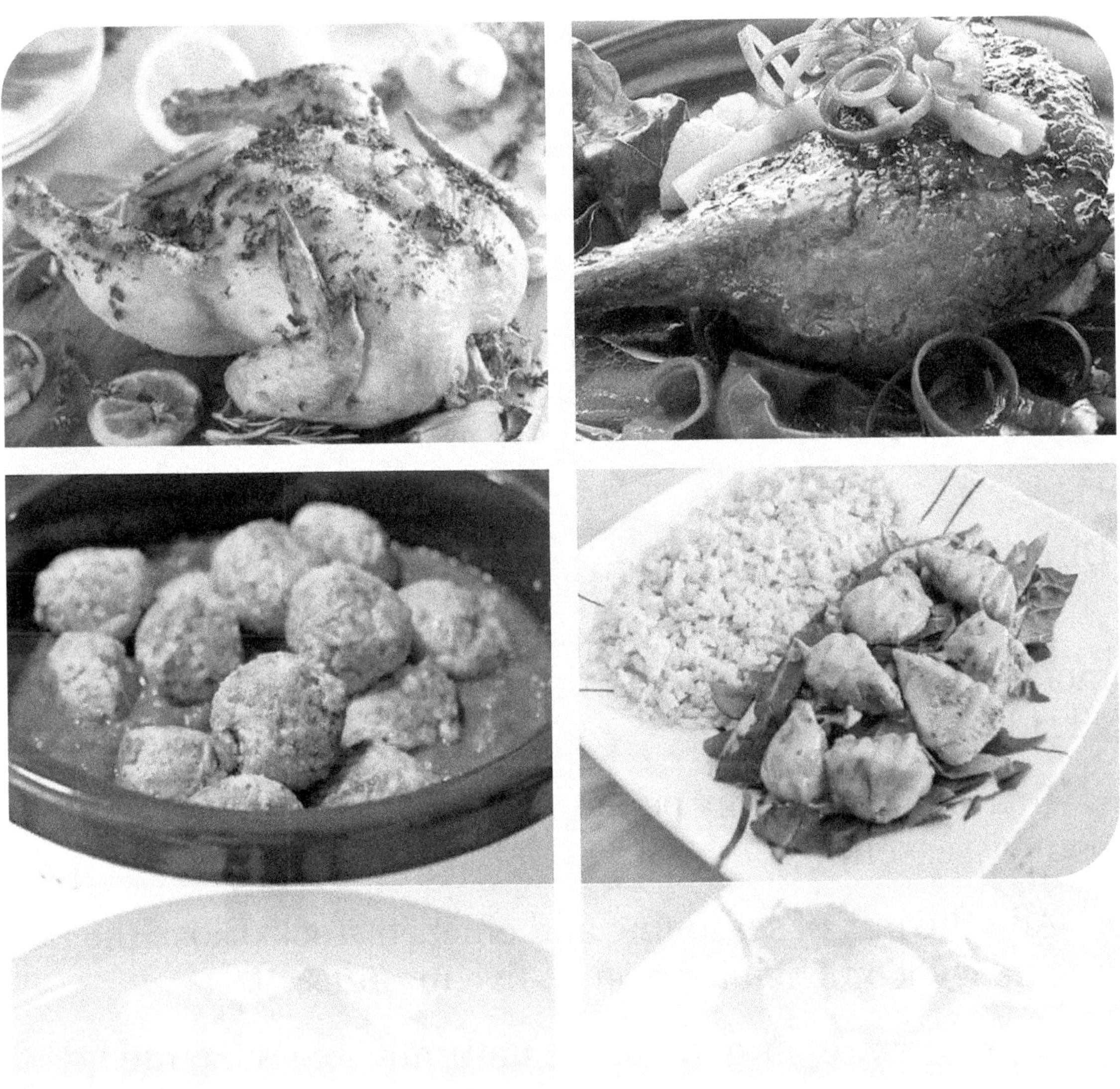

Time: 50 mins

Number of servings: 6

Ingredients:

Four-pound whole chicken

One tbsp coconut oil

Two cups chicken stock

One tsp paprika

A pinch of dried thyme

A pinch of poultry seasoning

Salt and pepper to taste

Directions:

•   Add coconut oil in your Instant Pot and select sauté mode. Then put a chicken in the pot. Cook until browned on all sides.

•   In a small bowl, mix pepper, paprika, salt, thyme, and poultry seasoning.

•   Add the mix of seasoning and chicken stock. Close the pot lid and cook on High for twenty-five minutes.

•   Allow the pressure to release naturally and open the lid. Serve and enjoy!

Time: 45 mins

Number of servings: 3

Ingredients:

Two pounds chicken thighs, boneless and skinless

Two cups brown rice, rinsed

Two cups sliced mushrooms

Two cups chopped carrots

One diced onion

Two cups chicken stock

Three minced cloves garlic

Two tbsp Worcestershire sauce

Two tbsp condensed cream of chicken soup

One tbsp fresh thyme

One tbsp olive oil

Salt and pepper to taste

Directions:

• Add olive oil in your Instant Pot and select sauté. Add onions and cook for three minutes.

• Now add rice, stock, veggies, and garlic. Place the chicken on top. Add salt and pepper. Pour the chicken with

Worcestershire sauce and chicken soup cream. Add thyme. Close the lid and cook on high for thirty minutes.

• Allow the pressure to release in a natural way and open the lid. Remove the springs and stir well. Serve and enjoy!

Simple Shredded Chicken

Time: 25 mins

Number of servings: 4

Ingredients:

One pound skinless and boneless chicken breast

One cup chunky salsa

One tsp cumin

A pinch of oregano

Salt and pepper to taste

Directions:

• Season chicken with cumin, salt, pepper, and oregano on both sides. Put seasoned poultry in your Instant Pot. Then pour chunky salsa on the chicken.

• Close the lid and select poultry mode. Cook for twenty five minutes then use rapid pressure release.

• Transfer chicken to a platter and shred it using two forks. Serve and enjoy!

Time: 45 mins

Number of servings: 4

Ingredients:

One pound lean ground turkey

Three cups sliced crimini mushrooms

Half cup long grain rice

One 24-oz can of pasta sauce

One chopped onion

Two sliced zucchini

Two tbsp minced Basil

Two tbsp olive oil

Half cup water

One tsp Italian seasoning

Salt to taste

Directions:

•   Add olive oil in your Instant Pot and select sauté mode. Add onion and cook for five minutes. Then add mushrooms, zucchini and cook for three minutes.

•   Add water and pasta, stir well. Continue cooking to bring it to a simmer.

- Meanwhile, in a bowl, mix ground meat, rice, and Italian herbs. Add salt and make 16 meatballs. Gently put these meatballs in the pot with boiling sauce.

- Close the lid and cook on high for twenty minutes. When ready, use rapid pressure release and open the lid. Sprinkle with basil and serve with your favorite garnish.

Time: 20 mins

Number of servings: 4

Ingredients:

One pound cut into cubes chicken breast, skinless and boneless

Two tbsp brown sugar

Two tbsp flour

One tbsp coconut oil

One tbsp ketchup

Half cup chicken stock

Three drops essential oil

Directions:

•   Put the meat and flour in one zip-lock bag and shake it to coat chicken well.

•   Add coconut oil in your Instant Pot and select sauté mode. Add chicken and cook for two minutes.

•   Now add stock, brown sugar, ketchup, orange essential oil and stir well. Close the lid and on high cook for fifteen minutes.

•   Use rapid pressure release and open the lid. Serve with your favorite garnish and enjoy!

Time: 30 mins

Number of servings: 3

Ingredients:

One pound chicken breast

One pound diced sweet potatoes

One chopped onion

Three tbsp butter

Three tbsp buffalo sauce

Half tsp onion powder

Half tsp garlic powder

Salt and pepper to taste

Directions:

• Add butter in your Instant Pot and select sauté mode. Add onions and cook for three minutes.

• Now add chicken, potatoes, buffalo sauce and spices. Close the lid and cook on high for eighteen minutes.

• Use rapid pressure release method and open the lid. Serve and enjoy!

Cheesy Lemon Chicken

Time: 20 mins

Number of servings: 3

Ingredients:

Three chicken breasts, boneless and skinless

Half cup crumbled feta cheese

One cup spicy salsa

Juice of one lemon

One tbsp olive oil

Half tsp chili powder

Half tsp ground cumin

Directions:

• Add oil in your Instant Pot and select sauté. Then add chicken and cook until brown on both sides.

• Remove chicken from the pot. Put in the pot salsa, chili powder, cumin, lime juice and stir well.

• Close the lid and cook on high pressure for eight minutes. Then use rapid pressure release and open the lid. Transfer meat with the sauce to a platter. Sprinkle with crumbled cheese, serve, and enjoy!

Time: 40 mins

Number of servings: 2

Ingredients:

Four small duck legs

Two cups sliced mushrooms

Four chopped pearl onions

One cup chicken stock

Half cup dry red wine

Two tbsp canola oil

Salt and pepper to taste

Directions:

• Add oil in your Instant Pot and select sauté mode. Rub salt with pepper onto the duck legs and transfer them to the pot. Cook until crispy brown.

• Remove the sautéed duck and extra fat from to a bowl and set aside. Reserve about three tbsp of the fat in the pot. Add mushrooms, onions, garlic, red wine and cook for five minutes.

• Now remove the sautéed mushrooms and set aside. Place sautéed duck in the pot and add chicken stock. Close the lid and cook on high for twenty five minutes.

- Use rapid pressure release and open the lid. Serve with the mushrooms and gravy.

Barbecue Chili Chicken

Time: 25 mins

Number of servings: 4

Ingredients:

One pound chicken thighs, boneless and skinless

One chopped onion

Quarter cup chili sauce

Quarter cup water

Two tbsp barbecue sauce

Two tbsp olive oil

One tbsp vinegar

Half tsp ground paprika

Salt and pepper to taste

Directions:

•   Add olive oil in your Instant Pot and select sauté. Then add chicken and cook until brown on both sides.

•   In a bowl, mix water, vinegar, onions, barbecue sauce, chili sauce, paprika, salt, and pepper. Pour that mixture over chicken.

•   Close the pot lid and cook on High for fifteen minutes. Then use rapid pressure release and open the lid. Serve hot and enjoy!

Time: 50 mins

Number of servings: 8

Ingredients:

Six and a half pounds turkey breast, skin-on and bone-in

One stalk celery, chopped

Two cups chicken stock

One onion, quartered

Three garlic cloves

Three tbsp cornstarch

Three tbsp cold water

Two tbsp butter

One sprig of thyme

One tsp paprika

One tsp onion powder

Salt and pepper to taste

Directions:

• Season turkey breast with spices and stuff with onion, garlic, celery, and thyme.

• Add butter in your Instant Pot and select sauté mode. Then add turkey breast and cook until brown.

- Now add chicken stock, close the lid and cook on high pressure for thirty-five minutes.

- Allow the pressure to release in a natural way and open the lid. Remove turkey, cover with foil and place on large plate.

- Whisk together cold water and cornstarch. Then add the mixture in the cooking pot. Select sauté mode and stir until broth thickened. Add salt and pepper.

- Slice the turkey, serve immediately and enjoy!

Time: 25 mins

Number of servings: 6

Ingredients:

Two chicken breasts, skinless and boneless

Six corn tortillas

One and a half cup tomato puree

Half cup water

Two diced onions

Two minced garlic cloves

Half tbsp cumin

Half tbsp dried and soaked ancho Chili

Half tsp salt

A pinch of chipotle powder

Directions:

•   In the blender, mix water, garlic, cumin, ancho Chili, chipotle powder, salt and puree them until smooth.

•   Pour that mixture into your Instant Pot. Add chicken, onions, tomato puree. Close the pot lid and cook on High for fifteen minutes.

- Use rapid pressure release and open the lid. Use the mixer to break up cooked chicken. Spoon taco and fill in the corn tortillas. Serve and enjoy!

Time: 60 mins

Number of servings: 3

Ingredients:

Two and a half pounds turkey quarters

Three pounds Yukon gold potatoes, halved

One chopped onion

Three minced garlic cloves

One chopped carrot

One stalk celery, chopped

Half cup grated Parmesan cheese

One cup chicken stock

Half cup milk

Two tbsp olive oil

Two tbsp butter

Three tbsp cornstarch

Two tbsp cold water

Two bay leaves

A pinch of dried sage

A pinch of dried rosemary

A pinch of dried thyme

Kosher salt and black pepper to taste

Directions:

•	Season turkey quarters with kosher salt and ground black pepper.

•	Add olive oil in your Instant Pot and select sauté mode. Place the seasoned turkey in the pot and brown each side for five minutes. Then remove and set aside.

•	Add in the pot onions and garlic and cook for two minutes. Then add carrots and celery and cook for five minutes. Now add bay leaves, rosemary, sage, thyme and sauté for another minute.

•	Add browned turkey and stock. Then place a steamer basket and add in potatoes. Close the lid and cook on high pressure for twenty minutes.

•	Allow the pressure to release in a natural way and open the lid. Remove the steamer basket and carefully place potatoes in a large bowl. Add milk, butter, Parmesan cheese. Mash potatoes and mix until smooth.

•	Remove the cooked turkey and set aside. Mix cornstarch and cold water in a small bowl. Stir the mixture into the turkey gravy and season with salt and pepper. Sprinkle the turkey gravy over mashed potatoes and turkey, serve and enjoy!

Time: 45 mins

Number of servings: 6

Ingredients:

One whole duck, chopped into chunks

Two diced green onions

One cubed potato

Four garlic cloves

One-inch piece fresh ginger root, sliced

Quarter cup water

Four tbsp soy sauce

Four tbsp sherry wine

Four tbsp sugar

Half tsp salt

Directions:

•   Place the chopped duck in your Instant Pot with skin side down and select sauté mode. Cook for ten minutes or until golden brown.

•   Add water, soy sauce, onion, garlic, ginger, sherry wine, salt, and sugar. Stir well, close the pot lid and cook on High for twenty minutes.

- Use rapid pressure release and open the lid. Add potato cubes, stir, close the lid and cook on high for another five minutes.

- Use rapid pressure release, open the lid, serve and enjoy!

Seafood is considered to be a good source of lean protein, Arginine, vitamin B1, B3, Biotin, B12. In fact, oily fish is the even more healthy option. The fatty skin of tuna and salmon contains vitamin D. Salmon is rich in vitamin A also. But the most significant health benefits lies in Omega-3 fatty acids. Eating oily fish can help to ease depression, reduce arthritis, and fight heart disease. Omega-3 fatty acids are good for your skin and eyes and have cancer-fighting properties.

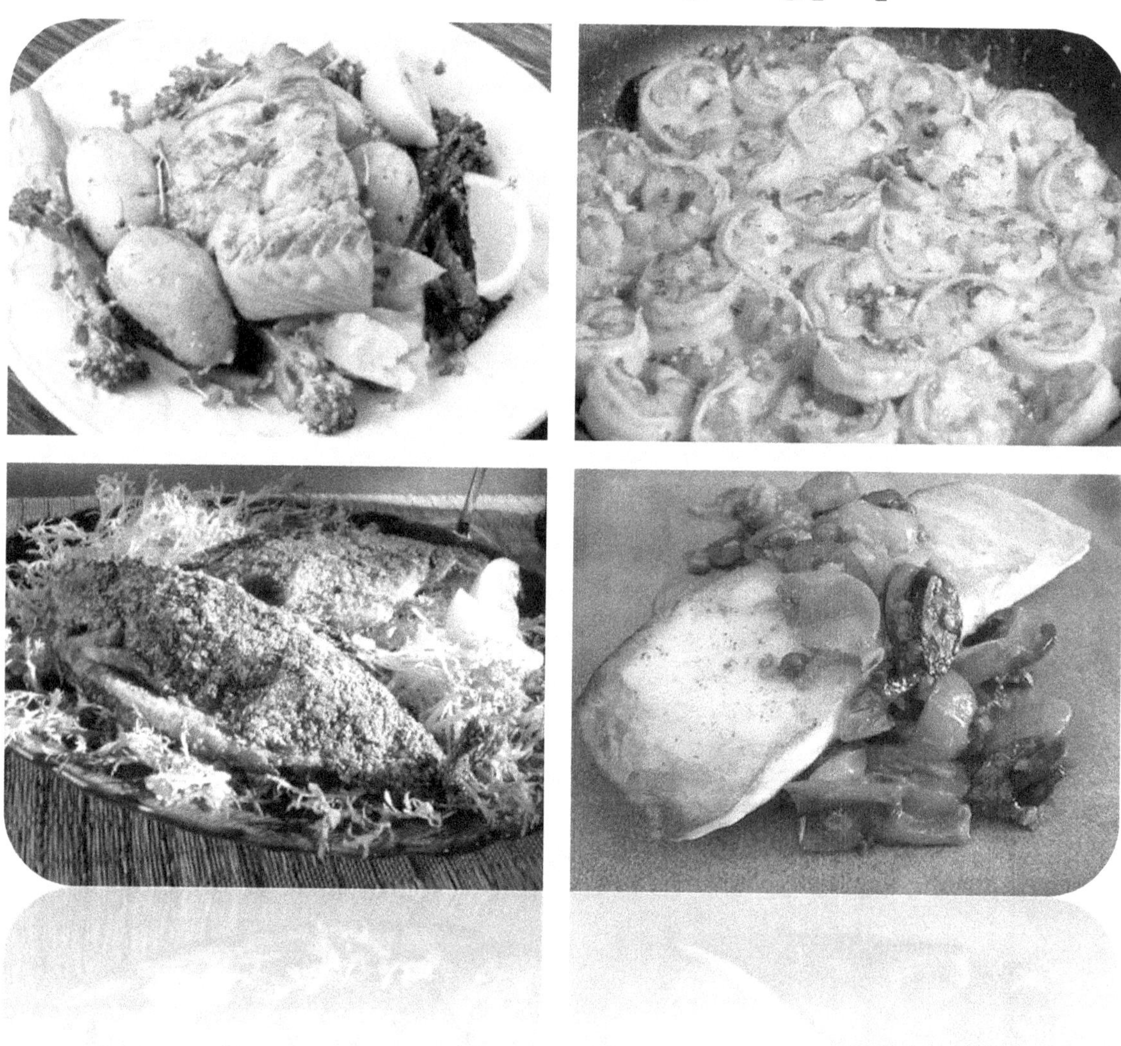

Time: 10 mins

Number of servings: 2

Ingredients:

One salmon fillet

Four new potatoes, cut in halves

Two cups broccoli florets

One tbsp butter

Herbs for seasoning

Salt and pepper to taste

Directions:

• Season the salmon, potatoes, and broccoli with salt, pepper, and herbs.

• Place a steamer basket and add in potatoes. Set it steam for about three minutes. Then use rapid pressure release.

• Put the salmon and broccoli florets in the basket and do the same for another three minutes.

• Allow the pressure to release in a natural way and open the lid. Place butter on the potatoes, serve and enjoy!

Time: 15 mins

Number of servings: 4

Ingredients:

Two pounds skinless halibut fillets

One chopped onion

Sixteen pitted and chopped green olives

Two 14-oz cans of diced tomatoes with juice

Two tbsp drained and chopped capers

Three tbsp minced pickled jalapeno rings

Two tbsp olive oil

Two tbsp lime juice

One tbsp minced garlic

Two sprigs oregano

Two sprigs rosemary

Directions:

•   Add olive oil in your Instant Pot and select sauté mode. Add garlic and onion and cook for two minutes.

•   Now add lime juice, jalapenos, olives, capers and herbs. Close the lid and cook on high for six minutes.

•   Use rapid pressure release and open the lid. Place fish right in the sauce. Close the lid and cook for another three minutes.

•   Use rapid pressure release again and open the lid carefully. Serve fish with the sauce and enjoy!

Time: 12 mins

Number of servings: 4

Ingredients:

Four salmon fillets

One lemon, sliced

Juice of one lemon

One cup water

Two tbsp chili pepper

Salt and pepper to taste

Directions:

•   Season salmon fillets with spices. Pour water in your Instant Pot. Place the steam rack in the pot and put the salmon in a single layer.

•   Close the lid and cook on high for six minutes. Then allow the pressure to release naturally and open the lid. Serve and enjoy!

Time: 10 mins

Number of servings: 4

Ingredients:

One pound frozen cod fillets

Two cups broccoli florets

One cup water

One tsp ginger

One tsp cumin

One tsp lemon pepper

Salt to taste

Directions:

• Cut fish into four pieces and season with salt, lemon pepper, cumin, and ginger.

• Pour a cup of water in your Instant Pot. Place the steam rack and put seasoned fish and broccoli in it. Close the lid and select chicken/meat mode. Cook for two minutes.

• Use rapid pressure release, open the lid, serve and enjoy!

Time: 25 mins

Number of servings: 4

Ingredients:

Two pounds shrimp, peeled and chopped

One peeled and minced onion

One peeled and minced shallot

Half celery stalk, minced

Four cups water

Half cup heavy cream

Three tbsp flour

Two tbsp tomato paste

Two tbsp butter

Three sprigs tarragon

Two sprigs thyme

Salt and pepper to taste

Directions:

• Add butter in your Instant Pot and select sauté mode. Add onion, shallot, celery, carrots and cook for four minutes. Then add flour and tomato paste and cook for two minutes.

- Now add water, herbs and select soup/stew mode. Cook for ten minutes then use rapid pressure release and open the lid.

- Add shrimp bits and cream. Select chicken/meat mode and simmer for two minutes. Season, serve, and enjoy!

Shrimp Scampi

Time: 20 mins

Number of servings: 4

Ingredients:

One pound frozen shrimp

One cup jasmine rice

Four minced garlic cloves

Two cups water

Quarter cup butter

Quarter cup chopped parsley

Juice of one lemon

A pinch of saffron

Salt and pepper to taste

Directions:

•   Place all ingredients except parsley in your Instant Pot. Stir well.

•   Close the lid and cook on high for ten minutes. Then use rapid pressure release.

•   Peel shells of shrimps, when you can touch them. Serve topped with parsley and enjoy!

•   Mix everything in your pressure cooker, leaving the shells on the shrimps.

Time: 30 mins

Number of servings: 4

Ingredients:

Two pounds peeled and deveined shrimp

Eight cut in quarters potatoes

One pound chopped tomatoes

Four chopped onions

Juice of one lemon

Four tbsp olive oil

One cup water

One tbsp watercress

One tsp curry powder

One tsp ground coriander

Salt to taste

Directions:

• Add water in your Instant Pot and place the steamer basket. Put potatoes in the steamer basket, close the lid and cook on high for ten minutes. Then use rapid pressure release, remove potatoes and set aside.

• Add oil in the pot and select sauté mode. Add onions, stir and cook for five minutes. Add curry, coriander, salt, stir and cook for another five minutes.

• Now add shrimp, tomatoes, lemon juice and cooked potatoes. Stir, close the lid and cook on high for three minutes.

• Release the pressure again, serve topped with watercress and enjoy!

Time: 15 mins

Number of servings: 4

Ingredients:

Two pounds trout fillets

Half cup sour cream

Three tbsp stone-ground mustard

One tbsp lemon juice

Lime wedges for garnish

Salt and pepper to taste

Directions:

- In a bowl, mix together salt, sour cream, mustard, lemon juice, and pepper. Spread the mixture over the fish with a spoon.

- Place the trout fillets in your Instant Pot. Close the lid and cook on high pressure for five minutes.

- Allow the pressure to release in a natural way and open the lid. Serve with lime wedges and enjoy!

Time: 20 mins

Number of servings: 4

Ingredients:

Four fillets codfish

One pound halved cherry tomatoes

One cup Taggiesche olives

Two minced garlic cloves

Two tbsp pickled capers

Two tbsp olive oil

Two sprigs thyme

Salt and pepper to taste

Directions:

•   Place tomatoes and olives in your Instant Pot. Add thyme and place the fish on top of the tomatoes.

•   Now add garlic, season with salt and pepper, sprinkle with the olive oil. Close the lid and cook at low pressure for seven minutes.

•   Allow the pressure to release naturally, serve and enjoy!

Time: 15 mins

Number of servings: 3

Ingredients:

One pound tilapia fillets

Three sliced scallions

Quarter cup soy sauce

Two tbsp olive oil

Three tbsp brown sugar

One tsp Chinese five-spice powder

Directions:

•   In a bowl, mix soy sauce and brown sugar. Season the fish with five-spice powder.

•   Add oil in your Instant Pot and select sauté. Place tilapia fillets and cook for two minutes, until they turn opaque.

•   Pour in the sauce mixture, close the lid and cook on high for five minutes.

•   Allow the pressure to release in a natural way and open the lid. Add scallions, serve warm and enjoy!

Pork Recipes

Lean pork can be an excellent addition to a healthy diet as it contains all the essential amino acids necessary for maintenance and muscle growth. In fact, high-quality protein is the main macronutrient of pork. Also, pork is rich in many healthy nutrients such as creatine, taurine, B vitamins, phosphorous, and selenium. Eating pork can help you to have a good immune to protect your body as well. Still, you need to consume pork in moderation because too much fat can be dangerous for you.

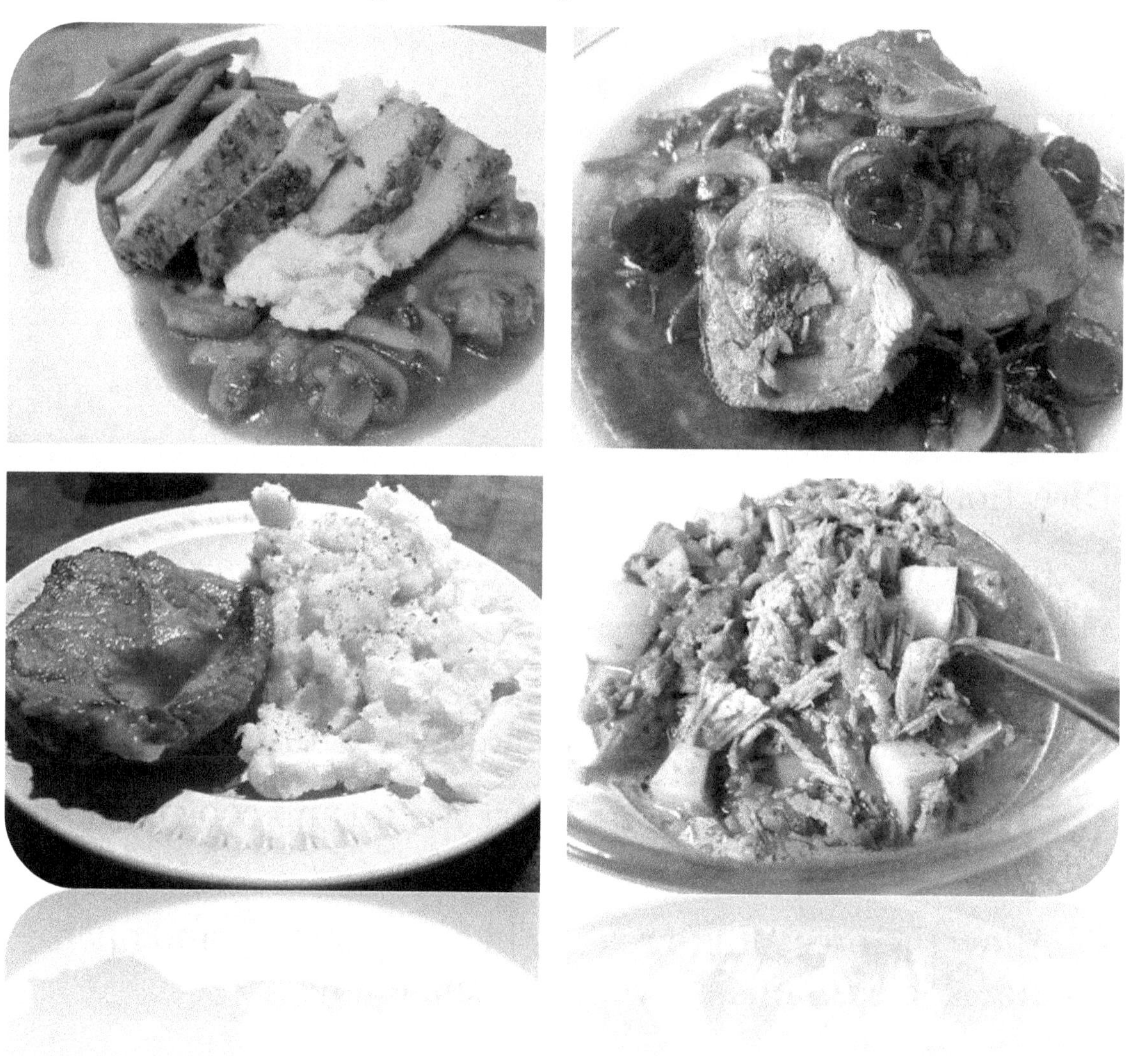

Time: 40 mins

Number of servings: 6

Ingredients:

Two pounds boneless pork chops

Two pounds chopped potatoes

One chopped yellow onion

Three minced garlic cloves

Two cups chicken stock

Two tbsp butter

Two tbsp white flour

One tsp smoked paprika

Mix of fresh herbs: sage, oregano, thyme, and rosemary

Salt and pepper to taste

Directions:

• Place potatoes in your Instant Pot. Add stock, onion, garlic, and herbs. Put pork chops on the top.

• Season with salt, pepper, and paprika. Close the pot lid and cook on high for fifteen minutes.

• Meanwhile, in a small pan, heat up butter. Add flour, and cook, stirring continuously, for two minutes and set aside.

- Use rapid pressure release and open the lid. Transfer pork to a platter and remove herbs.

- Transfer potatoes to a bowl. Add salt, pepper, and some cooking liquid. Stir with your hand mixer.

- Add butter-flour mix in a pot and select simmer mode. Cook stirring continuously, for two minutes, until it thickened.

- Serve pork chops, and mashed potatoes topped with the gravy from the pot and enjoy!

Time: 30 mins

Number of servings: 4

Ingredients:

One pound of pork sirloin tip roast, chopped into bite-sized pieces

One pound chopped sweet potato

One cup chopped fresh tomatoes

Two chopped onions

One 15-oz can of drained black beans

Half of 7-oz can diced green chilies

One cup chicken stock

Half cup chopped cilantro

One tbsp yogurt

One tbsp Italian seasoning

Half tbsp chili powder

One tbsp avocado oil

Salt and pepper to taste

Directions:

• Season meat with salt and pepper. Add oil in your Instant Pot and select sauté mode. Add meat, onions, chilies, chili powder, Italian seasoning and cook for two minutes.

• Now add stock, potatoes, black beans, and tomatoes. Close the lid and cook on high pressure for fifteen minutes.

• Use rapid pressure release, serve topped with yogurt and cilantro.

Time: 80 mins

Number of servings: 6

Ingredients:

Two pounds pork roast

Four cups chopped cauliflower

Two ribs celery, chopped

One chopped onion

Four minced garlic cloves

One 8-oz pack of portabella mushrooms, sliced

Two cups water

Two tbsp coconut oil

Salt and pepper to taste

Directions:

• Add onion, cauliflower, garlic, and celery to the bottom of your Instant Pot. Pour over water.

• Season pork roast with salt and pepper. Then place meat on the top of veggies. Close the lid and cook on high for sixty minutes.

• Use rapid pressure release, remove the pork and put it in an oven-proof dish. Bake at 400 degrees, until the edges are crisped.

•	Meanwhile, remove the stock and veggies and blend until smooth. Add mushrooms in your Instant Pot and sauté them for five minutes. Then add blended vegetables and cook for another five minutes.

•	Shred the meat, serve topped with mushroom gravy and enjoy!

Time: 50 mins

Number of servings: 4

Ingredients:

One and a half pound pork loin, boneless

Two cups chopped apple

Half cup chopped onion

Half cup pitted cherry

Half cup apple juice

Half cup chopped celery

One tbsp olive oil

Salt and pepper to taste

Directions:

• Place all ingredients mentioned above in your Instant Pot and stir well.

• Close the lid and select meat/stew mode. Cook for forty minutes.

• Use rapid pressure release, serve and enjoy!

Time: 30 mins

Number of servings: 2

Ingredients:

One cup pork loin chops, cut into 1-inch pieces

One cup long-grain rice

Half cup peas

One egg

Two carrots, chopped finely

One chopped onion

Two cups water

Four tbsp soy sauce

Two tbsp canola oil

Salt and pepper to taste

Directions:

•   Add oil in your Instant Pot and select sauté. Add onions, carrots and cook for four minutes.

•   Season meat with salt and pepper and add to the pot. Cook for eight minutes then transfer pork with veggies to a bowl.

•   Add rice and water in the pot. Close the pot lid and cook on High pressure for twenty minutes.

- Use rapid pressure release and open the lid. Spread rice, making the center of the pot vacant. Pour oil into the center, select sauté and add beaten egg.

- When the egg is almost cooked, add pork with vegetables and peas. Stir well, serve hot and enjoy!

Time: 70 mins

Number of servings: 4

Ingredients:

One pound pork shoulder blade, boneless and trimmed

One chipotle pepper

Three garlic cloves, cut into slivers

Half cup chicken stock

Two bay leaves

Half tsp cumin

A pinch of garlic powder

A pinch of dry oregano

A pinch of sazon

A pinch of dry adobo seasoning

Salt and pepper to taste

Directions:

•   Season meat with salt and pepper. In a pan, brown pork on all sides for five minutes on high heat. Then set aside to cool down.

•   Take a sharp knife and insert the blade into meat about 1-inch deep, then insert garlic slivers. You should do this on all sides of meat. Then season pork with cumin, garlic powder, adobo seasoning, oregano, and sazon.

•   Add stock, chipotle pepper and bay leaves in your Instant Pot. Stir well and add meat. Close the pot lid and cook on High for fifty minutes.

•   Allow the pressure to release in a natural way and open the lid. Shred pork with a couple of forks and mix it with juices. Remove bay leaves, serve hot and enjoy!

Time: 50 mins

Number of servings: 4

Ingredients:

Two pounds of pork loin roast, tied with kitchen string

Two and a half cups milk

Two tbsp butter

Two tbsp olive oil

One bay leaf

Salt and pepper to taste

Directions:

• Season meat with salt and pepper. Add butter in your Instant Pot and select sauté. Add olive oil and bay leaf. Place in meat, fat side down, and brown all over.

• Pour in milk, close the lid and cook on high for thirty minutes.

• Allow the pressure to release naturally and open the lid. Transfer the cooked meat to a platter and cover with foil.

• Remove the bay leaf from sauce in your Instant Pot and select sauté again. Cook, stirring continuously until you get desired thickness.

• Serve roast slices topped with sauce and enjoy!

Time: 30 mins, and 2 hours to marinate

Number of servings: 4

Ingredients:

Two pounds pork loin roast

Two sliced red onions

Six minced garlic cloves

One cup water

Half cup pineapple juice

Half cup soy sauce

Three tbsp canola oil

Two tbsp rice vinegar

Two tbsp brown sugar

One tbsp grated ginger

Directions:

•   Put pork, soy sauce, pineapple juice, half the garlic, ginger and brown sugar in one zip-lock bag and shake to coat meat well. Marinade for at least two hours.

•   In a skillet, cook marinated meat on a high heat until golden brown on all sides. Then set it aside.

•   Add oil in your Instant Pot and select sauté. Then add onions and cook for three minutes.

- Now add pork roast, marinade juices, water, and remaining garlic. Close the lid and cook on high pressure for twenty five minutes.

- Allow the pressure to release in a natural way and open the lid. Add rice vinegar and select sauté mode again. Simmer for ten minutes.

- Slice the meat, serve, and enjoy!

Time: 40 mins

Number of servings: 6

Ingredients:

Two pounds cubed stew pork

Two ounces diced pancetta

One chopped yellow onion

One diced carrot

Three minced garlic cloves

One 8-oz can of tomato sauce

One cup red wine

Two tsp Italian seasoning

One bay leaf

Salt and pepper to taste

Directions:

• Put pancetta in your Instant Pot and select sauté. Add the pork and cook until golden brown. Then add onions, carrots, garlic, red wine and cook for another two minutes.

• Now pour the tomato sauce over the meat. Add salt, pepper, Italian seasoning. Close the pot lid and cook on High for ten minutes.

- Use rapid pressure release. Remove bay leaf and stir well. Shred the meat with two forks. Serve with rice or pasta.

Time: 80 mins

Number of servings: 6

Ingredients:

Three pounds pork shoulder, cut into 1-inch cubes

Two pounds potatoes, peeled

One pound peeled and chopped carrots

Two onions, diced

One apple, peeled and diced

One 12-oz can of non-alcoholic cider

Half cup chopped parsley

One tbsp olive oil

Half tsp dried thyme

Half tsp dried sage

Salt and pepper to taste

Directions:

•   Season the meat with salt. Add olive oil in your Instant Pot. Brown the pork for three minutes per side. Transfer meat to a bowl and set aside.

•   Add onions and apple, stir, and cook for five minutes. Then add cider, bring to a boil, and boil for one minute.

•	Place the meat in the pot and stir well. Season with thyme and sage. Place a steamer basket in the pot and put the carrots and potatoes in the basket. Close the pot lid and cook on high for twenty-five minutes.

•	Allow the pressure to release naturally and open the lid. Serve topped with chopped parsley and enjoy!

Beef is a great source of various vitamins and minerals. B vitamins are vital for nervous system function, and rich store of zinc supports your immune system. Haem iron, the most absorbable form of iron would come from beef too. It builds your red blood cells and gives energy. Carnitine is another vital nutrient, which removes toxic compounds from cells and helps in our energy metabolism. The content of carnitine in seafood and poultry is low, however pretty high in beef.

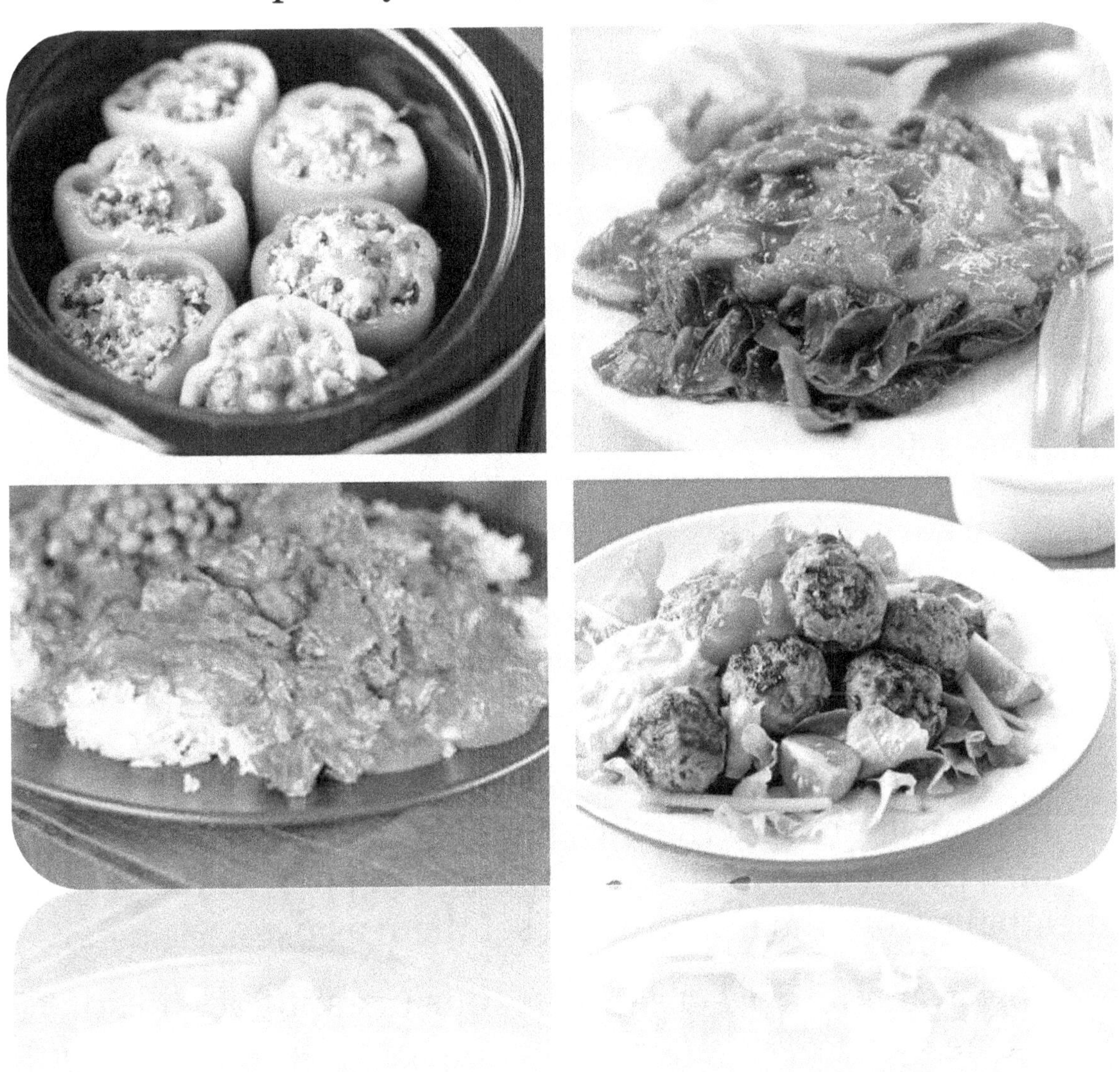

Time: 25 mins

Number of servings: 4

Ingredients:

One pound ground beef

Two chopped carrots

One chopped onion

One egg

Two slices of bread, crumbled

Two cup pasta sauce

Two cups water

Half tsp garlic powder

Salt and pepper to taste

Directions:

•   In a bowl, mix together ground beef, beaten egg, bread, onions, carrots, garlic powder, salt and pepper. Make meatballs from the mixture and set them aside.

•   Pour water and pasta sauce in your Instant Pot and stir well. One by one, add meatballs in the pot. Close the lid and cook on high pressure for six minutes.

•   Allow the pressure to release in a natural way and open the lid. Serve with rice or pasta and enjoy!

Time: 75 mins

Number of servings: 4

Ingredients:

Two pounds beef stew meat

One sliced green onion

Juice from one orange

Half cup soy sauce

Half cup water

Half cup brown sugar

Quarter cup sesame oil

One tbsp red pepper flakes

One tsp ginger powder

Half tsp garlic powder

Directions:

• In a bowl, mix together water, sesame oil, soy sauce, garlic powder, ginger powder, brown sugar, and pepper flakes. Add meat and marinate for thirty minutes.

• Transfer everything from the bowl into your Instant Pot. Add orange juice, close the lid and select stew/meat. Cook for thirty five minutes.

- Use rapid pressure release and open the lid. Top beef with green onions, serve with rice and enjoy!

Time: 35 mins

Number of servings: 4

Ingredients:

One pound ground beef

One cup brown rice

One cup crumbled mozzarella cheese

Four large bell peppers

One 8-oz can of tomato sauce

One diced tomato

One chopped onion

One egg

Half tsp garlic powder

Half tsp oregano

Half tsp dried parsley

Salt and pepper to taste

Directions:

• In a bowl, mix together tomato, ground beef, rice, egg, oregano, parsley, onions, salt, and pepper.

• With a sharp knife slice off the bell peppers tops. Then stuff the bell peppers with the ground meat mixture.

•   Pour water and half of tomato sauce in your Instant Pot. Then place a trivet in the pot and put stuffed peppers on the trivet. Pour remaining tomato sauce over peppers. Close the pot lid and cook on high for fifteen minutes.

•   Allow the pressure to release naturally and open the lid. Serve topped with mozzarella cheese and enjoy!

Time: 60 mins

Number of servings: 4

Ingredients:

Two pounds boneless beef chuck shoulder roast, trimmed of fat and cut into 2-inch cubes

One finely chopped onion

Four sliced shallots

Two minced garlic cloves

Half cup pitted and chopped Medjool dates

Half cup beef stock

Half cup chopped parsley

Quarter cup balsamic vinegar

Quarter cup red wine

Two tbsp olive oil

Three tbsp flour

Half tsp dried oregano

Salt and pepper to taste

Chopped parsley for garnish

Directions:

- Put beef, flour, oregano, salt, and pepper in one zip-lock bag and shake to coat meat well.

- Add olive oil in your Instant Pot and select sauté mode. Then add seasoning meat, onion, shallots, garlic, and cook, stirring occasionally, for five minutes.

- Now add stock, wine, balsamic vinegar and stir well. Close the lid and cook on high for forty minutes.

- Allow the pressure to release in a natural way and open the lid. Serve topped with chopped parsley and enjoy!

Spicy Braised Beef

Time: 80 mins

Number of servings: 4

Ingredients:

Two pounds eye of round beef, trimmed of fat and cut into 3-inch pieces

Four cloves garlic

Half of onion

Juice of one lemon

Two tbsp chipotle peppers in adobo sauce

One cup water

One tbsp olive oil

One tbsp ground oregano

One tbsp ground cumin

Two tsp kosher salt

A pinch of ground cloves

Three bay leaves

Black pepper to taste

Directions:

• Season the beef with salt and pepper. Add oil in your Instant Pot and select sauté mode. Place meat in the pot and cook it until golden brown.

• Meanwhile, in your blender, combine water, lime juice, chipotle peppers, onion, garlic, cloves, and oregano.

• Pour that blended mixture in the pot. Add bay leaves, close the lid and cook on high pressure for one hour.

• Allow the pressure to release naturally and open the lid. Remove bay leaves. Transfer cooked meat to a platter and shred it with two forks. Serve shredded beef with sauce from the pot and enjoy!

Time: 60 mins

Number of servings: 4

Ingredients:

Two pounds flank steak

Half cup olive oil

Quarter cup of apple cider vinegar

Two tbsp onion soup mix

One tbsp Worcestershire sauce

Directions:

• Add olive oil in your Instant Pot and select sauté mode. Add the steak and cook until browned.

• Add vinegar, Worcestershire sauce, and soup mix. Close the pot lid and cook on high for thirty-five minutes.

• Use rapid pressure release and carefully open the lid. Serve with your favorite garnish and enjoy!

Time: 50 mins

Number of servings: 4

Ingredients:

Two pounds boneless beef

Ten potatoes, peeled and chopped

Six chopped carrots

Two chopped onions

Two cups hot water

Two tbsp onion soup mix

Directions:

• In a bowl, mix together hot water and onion soup mix. Place the beef in your Instant Pot and pour onion soup mixture over the meat.

• Add potatoes, onions, carrots and stir well. Close the lid and select meat/stew mode. Cook for forty minutes.

• Use rapid pressure release and carefully open the lid. Serve hot and enjoy!

Time: 75 mins

Number of servings: 6

Ingredients:

Two pounds chuck steak

Half pound sliced white button mushrooms

One sliced onion

Three minced garlic cloves

One cup chicken stock

One cup sour cream

Half cup dry white wine

Half cup chopped parsley

Two tbsp cornstarch

Two tbsp cold water

One tbsp olive oil

One tbsp flour

Salt and pepper to taste

Directions:

- Season meat with salt and pepper. Add oil in your Instant Pot and select sauté. Place beef in the pot and cook for seven minutes on each side. Then transfer meat to a platter and set aside.

- Add mushrooms and sauté them for eight minutes. Now add onion and garlic and cook for another two minutes. Pour in wine and allow it to reduce for two minutes.

- Meanwhile, cut the chuck steak into thin slices. In a bowl, mix beef slices with flour. Add meat and chicken stock in the pot. Close the lid and cook on high for twelve minutes.

- Allow the pressure to release in a natural way and open the lid. Select sauté and slowly pour sour cream in the pot while stirring.

- Mix cornstarch and cold water in a small bowl. Add the mixture to the pot and stir well. Top with chopped parsley, serve with favorite garnish and enjoy!

Lamb Recipes

Lamb is a red meat, so in moderation, this meat is an excellent source of protein, vitamin B12, selenium, and iron. Usually, lamb has less marbling of fat within so you can trim most of the fat easily. Lamb is also a good source of immune-boosting zinc. This nutrient aids wound healing, supports the immune system, optimizes protein synthesis and maintains healthy testosterone levels.

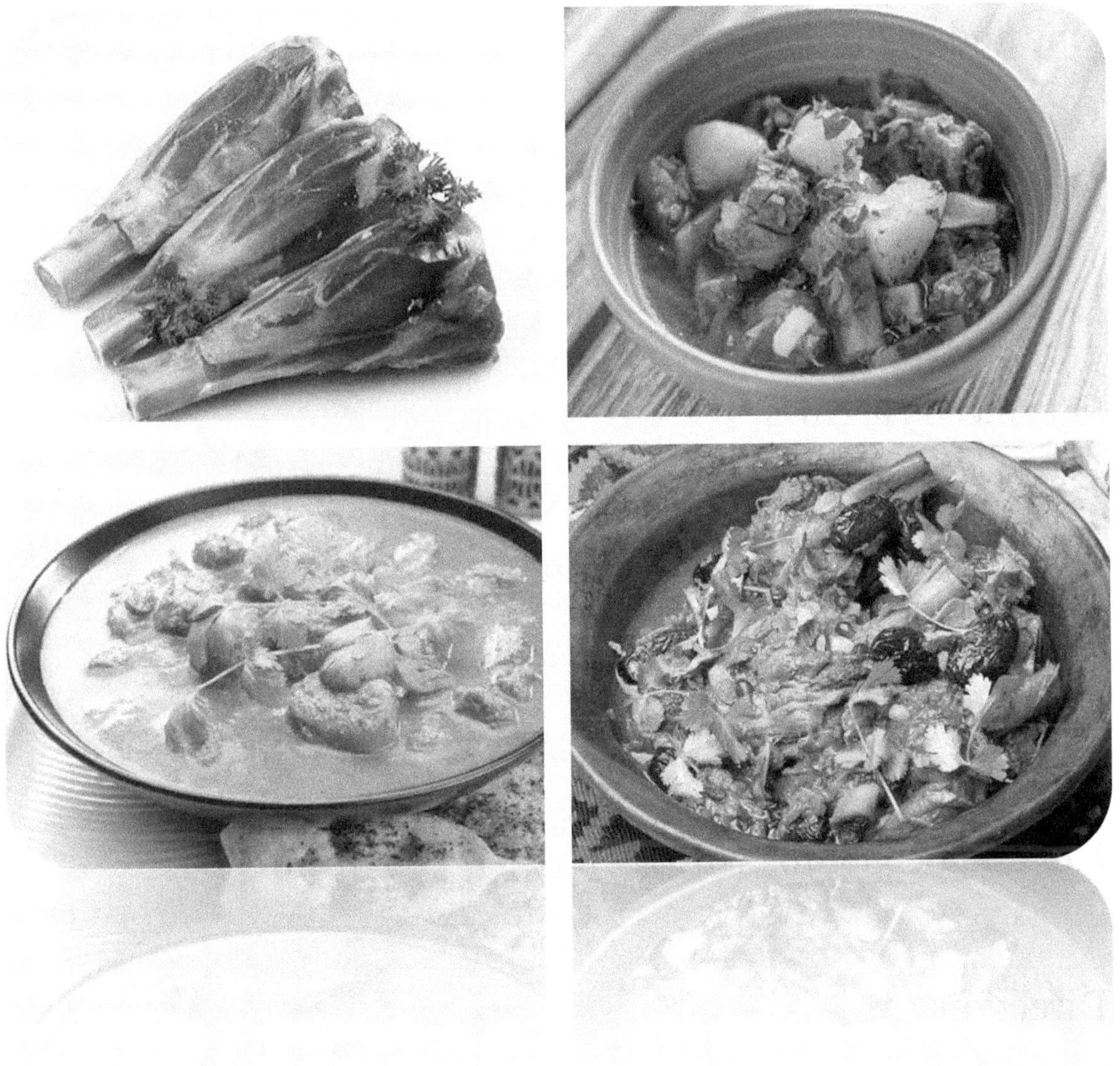

Time: 35 mins

Number of servings: 4

Ingredients:

One and a half pounds of lamb stew meat, cubed

One 15-oz can of diced tomatoes

One chopped onion

Four minced garlic cloves

Three chopped carrots

One diced zucchini

1-inch piece of fresh ginger, grated

Half cup coconut milk

Juice of half lemon

One tbsp butter

One tbsp curry powder

Salt and pepper to taste

Directions:

• Put meat, lime juice, coconut milk, garlic, ginger, salt, and pepper in one zip-lock bag and shake to coat meat well. Marinate in refrigerator for at least thirty minutes.

- Put the lamb with marinade in your Instant Pot. Add tomatoes with juice, butter, onions, carrots, and curry powder. Close the lid and cook on high for twenty minutes.

- Allow the pressure to release in a natural way and open the lid. Select sauté mode, add zucchini and simmer for six minutes. Serve over rice and enjoy!

Time: 120 mins

Number of servings: 4

Ingredients:

Two pounds leg of lamb

One sliced red onion

Eight whole garlic cloves, peeled

Seven dried dates

One cup chicken stock

One tbsp tomato paste

One tbsp coconut oil

One tbsp balsamic vinegar

One tbsp corn starch

One tbsp cold water

Three bay leaves

One tsp cinnamon

One tsp ginger powder

One tsp turmeric powder

One tsp ground coriander seed powder

One tsp ground cumin

Salt and pepper to taste

Directions:

• Season the lamb leg with salt, pepper, coriander seed, turmeric, and cumin powder. Add coconut oil in your Instant Pot and select sauté mode.

• Add the leg of lamb and cook for three minutes on each side. Then add onions and ginger. Sauté each side for one minute, stirring onions and ginger.

• Add stock, vinegar, tomato paste, garlic, dates, cinnamon, and bay leaves in the pot. Stir well, close the pot lid and cook on High pressure for eighty minutes.

• Use rapid pressure release and carefully open the lid. Transfer the lamb to a platter. Then select sauté again and let the sauce in the pot bubble away for ten minutes.

• Meanwhile, cut the lamb meat away from the bone and shred it with two forks. Mix together cornstarch with cold water, then add the mixture to the pot and stir well.

• Remove bay leaves and add the lamb back in the pot. Serve with your favorite garnish and enjoy!

Time: 90 mins

Number of servings: 6

Ingredients:

Two pounds lamb meat, trimmed of fat and cut into cubes

Six red potatoes, sliced

Three peeled and sliced carrots

Two chopped leeks

Two chopped onions

One chopped turnip

Two minced garlic cloves

Two tbsp olive oil

Four cups chicken stock

One 12-oz bottle dark beer

Half cup chopped parsley

One tbsp dried thyme

Two bay leaves

Salt and pepper to taste

Directions:

• Season the meat with dried thyme, salt, and pepper. Add olive oil in your Instant Pot and select sauté. Then add the lamb and cook until brown. Then transfer to a platter and set aside.

• Now add onions and sauté for three minutes. Add garlic and cook for another one minute. Add the meat back in the pot and stir well.

• Pour in stock and beer, close the lid and cook on high for thirty minutes.

• Allow the pressure to release in a natural way and open the lid. Add potatoes, turnips, carrots, leeks and bay leaves. Stir well, close the pot lid and cook on high for ten minutes.

• Use rapid pressure release and carefully open the lid. Remove bay leaves. Serve topped with fresh chopped parsley and enjoy!

Thank you for getting this book. Now you know that you do have the power to change your life. I hope that you will use these information, tips, and recipes to achieve your health goals. Always be sure that you are eating whole foods, keeping track of physical activity, and drinking enough water.

Coordinate with your doctor when changing your eating plan or starting a new type of fitness training. It's especially important if you have any metabolic, heart, or other conditions that may impact on your diet and exercise routine.

It is a well-known fact that one of the best ways of losing excess weight is to eat more homemade meals that utilize fresh and whole foods. By doing so, you increase intake of nutrients, which are highly beneficial to your health, like fiber, protein, complex carbohydrates, good fats, vitamins, and minerals. At the same time, making your meals allows you to cut back on sugar, salt, trans-fats, food additives, and preservatives.

Thanks again for reading this book! Eat healthily and think positively!

Meal Prep with Oven-Baked Recipes

Introduction

You don't have to eat less. You just have to eat right!

It's a well-known fact that proper nutrition is a crucial point for our general health. Ideally, we want to eat home cooked whole foods with enough variety to provide us with all needed nutrients. However, who has time to prepare food every day in our busy lives?

Thanks to meal prep, you can eat delicious food and maintain a balanced, healthy diet. Also, you will learn how to save both of your precious things – your time and your money by mastering the food-prepping process. Indeed, having a food prep container filled with your favorite healthy meal saves your minutes and your dollars. Moreover, it eliminates the stress of figuring out what to eat every single time. You don't have to worry about your cravings and going out to eat when you're working. Meal prep makes your healthy living so easy that it fills like a magic!

Don't be afraid to start small; you should build your own meal prep gradually, without getting overwhelmed. Even just prepping lunches or snacks will be a great beginning! What's your schedule look like? At least, you should be eating a breakfast, lunch, and dinner. Obviously, it's all about finding a healthy balance as with everything else in our life.

Never force yourself to eat certain health foods if you don't like them. Instead, choose healthy versions of the foods you like, such as spiralized veggie noodles as an alternative to pasta. Anyway, there is a wide variety of healthy foods to choose from so you definitely can enjoy the health advantages of whole foods without compromising on taste and flavor.

Good carbs found in whole grains, lean proteins, and fruits with vegetables are the way to go to maintain a well-balanced whole foods diet. Personally, I don't calculate exact numbers of macronutrients, and my usual meal consists of 1 part protein, 1 part carbs, and 2 parts veggies. Sure thing, you can alter this depending on your goals.

In fact, preparing food a couple of times per week can be pleasing and even entertaining which is opposite to cooking every single night. Meal prep involves planning the meals ahead of time, shopping, batch cooking and then stocking your fridge with various healthy meals, including snacks. Later in this book, we will anatomize each and every step of this amazing food prep process. And right now, we are going to focus on meal prep benefits.

Eat healthy, live longer!

Time savings

Meal prep gives you more time in the evenings to relax, work out, or do whatever you want. You have options other than rushing home to cook, and it is possible due to the cooking in bulk. Also, having things ready to go helps you save time worrying about food and ordering food during the work week. Imagine only on Sunday night you go to sleep knowing that you are set for the next few days or an entire week. In fact, food prep does not have to be an entire week; it works for you according to your schedule.

Money Saving

Meal prep helps you save your money by budgeting your grocery shopping and by not eating out. Well, we all know that dining out is expensive. Naturally, you save a significant amount of money, preparing most of your meals at home.

Batch cooking allows you to purchase more discounted bulk ingredients. As a result, you will save your money. Even more, you can base your week meal plan on what is on sale. In this case, you should plan your recipes only after grocery shopping. Eventually, you will buy fresh foods and spend less money on food. And your menu is variable enough because sales change every week. Just think about it.

Also, food prep helps to reduce the amount of food waste. Just because you plan your meals ahead, you are significantly less likely to throw out food than other people.

Food variety

When you prepare a bunch food in advance, you will have a lot of the same food, which can get a little monotonous. By focusing on cooking ingredients rather than meals, you can avoid getting bored at consuming the same thing every day. Use your ingredients in different combinations to get an assortment of go-to recipes that you can rotate throughout the week.

It's a good practice to try at least one new recipe each week. Change up different cultures, spices, and flavors to reduce food fatigue and keep it fresh. Most people follow the same routine and eat the same meals every day for years without even realizing it. Meal prep will open the fun world of food to you!

Healthier eating

Food prep helps you to get control over both the ingredients and your personal portion size. When you fueled your body with the healthiest whole foods you can possibly find, you want to work out much more.

You should not make any food choices when you're in a rush, hungry or just feeling lazy. Having your healthy meals at the ready means, you're far less tempted to eat fast-food, sweets and junk. Instead of relying on your willpower, which in most cases will fail you, meal prep allows us to plan healthy food ahead of time.

Portion control

It is a well-known fact that control of your portion sizes is the key to weight loss. But eating out and your portion control do not mix well at all. Restaurants just sell the same portion size of their dishes to every client. And meal prepping provides you with instant portion control.

To figure out your optimal portion size, make notes of how you feel after the meal and what sizes worked best for you. You should feel satisfied enough without putting yourself in a food coma. Buy the food containers of appropriate size, and you will be less likely to overeat. In the next chapter, we will consider your food containers in more detail.

And of course, if you want to lose weight, use portion sizes a bit smaller than you'd usually have and eat more non-starchy vegetables.

Consistency

Meal prepping makes consistency a lot easier since you can answer the question "What's for dinner tonight?" without any stress. You simply do not have to worry about it because it is already done. It is consistency at its finest, isn't it?

You don't have to cook thirty meals in one day to feel the benefits of food prep. If you try to prepare too much too soon, you may end up feeling overwhelmed and wasting your food. Start small and triple your favorite whole foods recipe so you can have it several times throughout the week. Your success positively will motivate you to keep going. When you see your bank account and your body change, you will naturally start to enjoy meal prep even more. It's one of the healthiest habits you can develop.

Obviously, you need some meal prep containers, if you want your food transfer to be easy. As you already know, the size matters. I mean you should found your perfect portion size and stick to it in order to avoid feeling unsatisfied or binge eating. Eating the right portions is an equally crucial thing for losing, maintaining or gaining weight. Feel free to experiment with container sizes before purchasing a set so you can figure out your proper meal portion size.

High-quality containers last a long time; they are durable, airtight, fridge friendly, BPA free, microwave and dishwasher safe. If you are serious about food prep, investing in a few superior containers will save your money and simplify the process significantly.

Food prep containers with dividers are helpful for portioning out your protein, carbohydrates, and vegetables. And if you didn't want certain foods to touch, this option is for you too.

Small sized containers are ideal to keep snacks because you can take it in your handbag when you are on the go. And glass jars could be used for storing oats, muesli, salads, desserts, smoothies, and juices.

The amount of containers you need depends on how many meals you are going to prep per week. For entire work week, you should have, at very least, five containers for lunch and five containers for dinner. And add two extra just in case.

Failing to plan is a planning to fail!

Naturally, when it comes to meal prep, planning is the key factor. Meal planning allows you to make all healthy decisions for the week in one sitting. So in the middle of the work week, you can focus on your tasks thoroughly since you don't have to worry about being healthy. At the same time, it's not a simple and easy thing to get right the first time. But don't worry about it – you will do better next time.

For the first month, you should work your food prep into your routine. So it is clever to schedule off a block of meal prepping time so that it falls on certain days of the week. If your work timetable allows, you can do it twice a week. Anyway, you will need enough time to peel, slice, cook, and store all planned foods. In most cases, four hours are enough for prepping meals for an entire week. And it will be only two hours if you split the process to two days a week. Keep things organized, and you will do the easiest and quickest prep.

Even if you have only a few ideas for dinner, your weekly meal plan helps organize grocery shopping so you can save time and money and reduce food waste. A healthy lifestyle doesn't have to be too hard to maintain. Firstly, you have to commit to it in your mind and then plan the rest out from there. And so the next thing you need to do is make a list of your favorite healthy recipes you can depend on. Over time, you will find a core set of dishes that you know works. Versatile enough meal plan that can be used as your go-to for the months makes the food prep routine much easier.

The best thing about your **individual meal plan** is that you can incorporate your schedule and avoid prepping more meals than you need on a work week. Every week is different and this way you can take into consideration your travel, date, and days you will buy lunch at work. So take a look at your weekly schedule and **count the meals** you need to prep at home. We don't know how much food to purchase unless we look at how many meals we want to make.

	Monday	Tuesday	Wednesday	Thursday	Friday
Breakfast					
Lunch					
Snack					
Dinner					

Now decide on your dishes and write down some options for breakfast, lunch, and dinner. You should plan and cook foods you actually enjoy eating. Make sure each your meal includes a balance of vegetables, complex carbohydrates, and lean protein. Eating the same dish every single day could be boring, but you can make several different meals with a limited number of ingredients. Answer these questions in order to define your desires and possibilities:

•   What did you have last week? And what are you craving this week?

•   What vegetables and fruits are in season?

•   What meat and fish are on sale?

•   What new recipe do you want to try?

Don't choose a recipe that requires a small amount of a new for you ingredient you will never use again. Or you can try to substitute this component with a more typical product. For example, you can replace coconut milk with Greek yogurt or condensed cow milk. Contrariwise, you are going to end up throwing some of the purchased foods right in the garbage.

Before making a grocery list check your pantry, freezer, and fridge for what you need. Without this step, you are going to end up with way too much of some products. You can also correct this week's menu according to available ingredients and previously frozen meals.

Finally, make your shopping list based on the disposition of food categories in your grocery store. **Put your ingredients on the list in a particular order in which they follow each other when you walk through the store.** This way you will save your precious time and won't forget stuff on your list.

If you keep whole foods in your fridge,

You will eat whole foods!

Now it is time to go **shopping**. Don't buy on impulse and avoid soda and sugary snacks. Instead, buy fruits that are in season at the moment. Usually, they are on sale. Look for fruits and veggies that have deep colors and look heavy for their size to get the juiciest, ripest and most nutrition-packed foods.

When it comes to buying in bulk, consider which wholesale club works best for you and use it as much as possible. This way cooking in bulk saves you money. Stuff like whole grains, lentils, pasta, nuts, and seeds can last long periods of time in your pantry so don't be afraid to buy them in bulk. You can also stock your freezer with meat, fish, vegetables, fruits, and berries. By the way, some frozen foods can pack more nutrients than actually fresh. And it is a life-saving hack if sometimes you just have no time for shopping.

Canned meat, fish, beans, and tomatoes are great for some recipes. They also can sit in your pantry for months and be used when you need last-minute food prep. But please don't eat canned foods all the time!

Store ethylene-producing fruits and veggies such as tomatoes, bananas, pears, and avocados separately from ethylene-sensitive potatoes, apples, carrots, and broccoli. Also, ensure that plants are completely dry before you store them because they spoil much faster if stored wet. Remember that plant foods with higher water content like cucumbers won't store as long as something like potatoes.

The lower shelves of your fridge provide proper storage for your veggies and fruits.

On the flip side, top shelves provide the best place for cooked meals. If you are prepping on Sunday the meal that you plan to eat on Friday, put it in your freezer and defreeze it in the fridge Thursday night. So, if you plan to cook only one day during the week, you should schedule freezer-friendly dishes at the end of the week. Don't forget that some foods such as sweet potatoes and eggs do not freeze well.

Love yourself enough to eat healthy!

If you have two days for meal prep, cook the more complicated dishes on the weekend day. Cooking less complicated meals during your mid-week meal prep day helps to save energy and enthusiasm. Your oven, Crockpot or Instant Pot are just great time savers since you need just add ingredients and set it. While it is cooking one recipe, you have time to prepare another.

As a rule, meat takes a while to cook which provides you with time to get other stuff done. So, it's natural enough to cook in the following sequence: meat, carbohydrates, and vegetables. You should write down or set timers, so you will know how long everything has been preparing. Cooking several compatible ingredients gives you the flexibility to mix them together easily in a variety of ways to create quick, healthy and tasty meals. For example, baked poultry without any skin is easy enough to reheat and pair with whole grains, new sauces, and greens. You can also use it to make salad, sandwiches, or pizza.

And you can even make your own healthy minute whole grain meals. For this, cook in bulk quinoa or brown rice and cool it in your fridge. Then divide the cooked grains into meal-size containers to freeze. Now you may reheat and enjoy it anytime.

Chop and slice your veggies according to the recipe ahead of time. This way you will cut cooking time in half. Also, having chopped fruits and vegetables stimulates you to eat more salads and plant-based snacks. As a result, you will less tend to eat things like ice cream, candy bars, or doughnuts.

As lean meat, poultry is rich in protein and contains less amount of fat. Protein promotes growth and repair in your body. Also, protein helps you feel full for a more extended period of time after a meal.

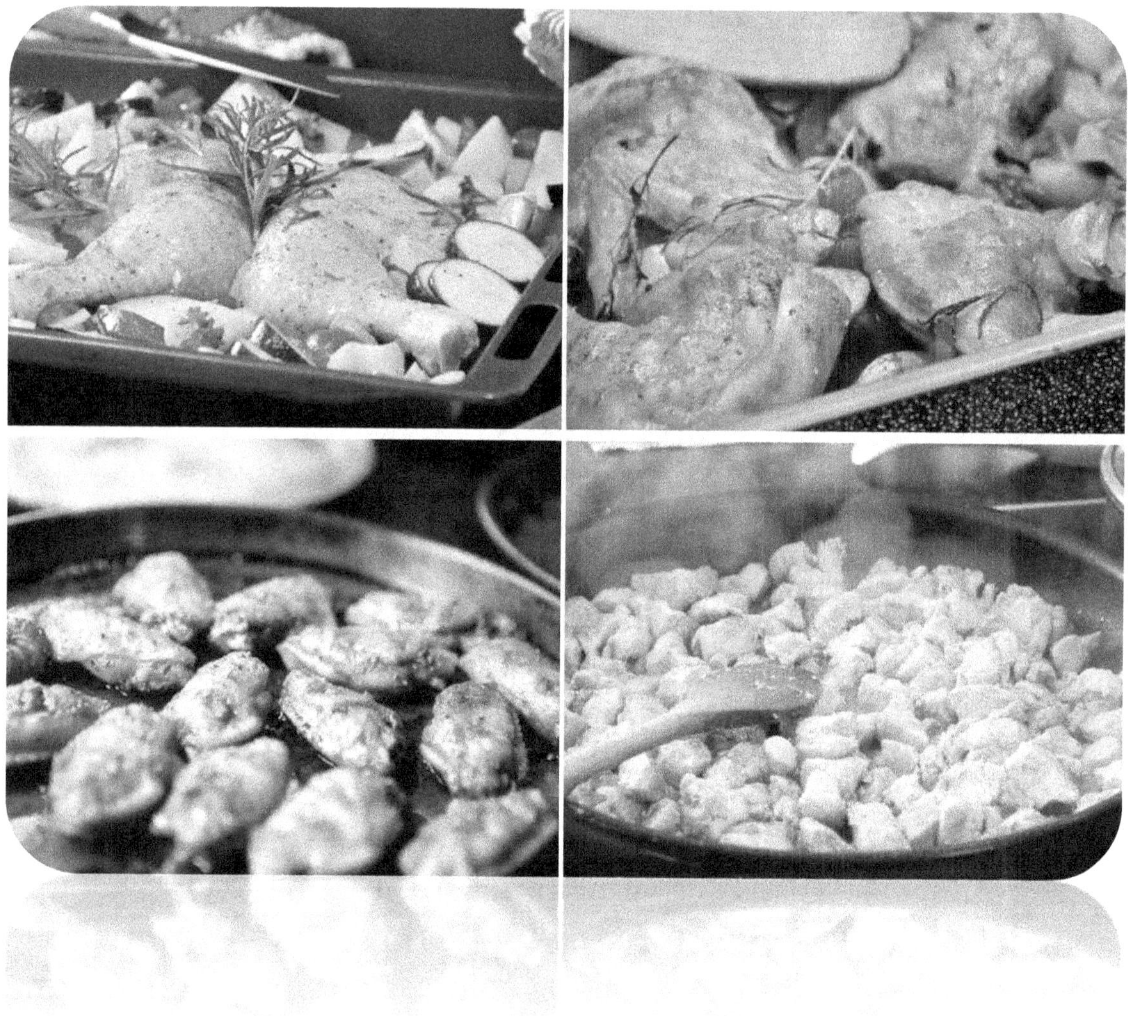

Besides protein, poultry contains several essential for our health vitamins and minerals. Poultry, being rich in B vitamins, maintain your skin health, nervous system, vision, and digestive system. Vitamin B6 and Niacin play an enormous role in preventing heart disease development.

Poultry intake aids in strong bones and teeth since it contains phosphorous and calcium. Phosphorous maintains healthy bones and teeth and improves the functioning of central nervous system, liver, and kidneys. Poultry also has selenium which is known to cut the risk of arthritis, improving metabolism, and regulating body weight.

Poultry is an excellent source of zinc which is essential for your immune system, wound healing, and hormonal balance. Notably, men should eat foods rich in zinc to regulate testosterone levels and boost the production of sperms.

Consuming poultry enhances your mood, acting as a natural anti-depressant. It contains two nutrients that are helpful for reducing stress – Vitamin B5 and Tryptophan. Tryptophan is an amino acid which increases the level of Serotonin. Also, Serotonin is one of the neurotransmitters that control depression and minimize stress.

Time: 60 mins

Number of servings: 3

Ingredients:

One pound chicken breast, cut into bite-sized pieces

One cup rice

One cup chopped lettuce

One cup feta cheese

Half cup halved olives

One chopped into wedges lemon

Juice of one lemon

One chopped red pepper

Half onion, chopped

One minced garlic clove

Two Tbsp olive oil

One tsp cumin

One tsp oregano

Salt and pepper to taste

Directions:

•   In a bowl, mix together the juice of lemon, one Tbsp olive oil, garlic, oregano, salt, and pepper. Place the chicken in a plastic zip-lock bag and add the prepared marinade. Toss to coat and place in the refrigerator for forty minutes.

•   Meanwhile, cook the rice according to the info on the package and add the cumin.

•   In a large skillet, heat up the remaining Tbsp olive oil over medium heat. Add the marinated chicken pieces and cook for three minutes per side.

•   When rice is cooked, divide it into the three containers. Add chicken, feta, olives, onions, peppers, and lettuce to each bowl. Top with lemon wedges and let your prepped meals cool down before storing in your fridge.

Time: 45 mins

Number of servings: 3

Ingredients:

One pound chicken breast, sliced

One cup brown rice

Four chopped red peppers

One chopped onion

One Tbsp olive oil

One tsp cumin

One tsp oregano

Half tsp garlic powder

Half tsp cayenne pepper

Salt and pepper to taste

Directions:

- Preheat your oven to 350°F.

- Cook the brown rice according to the info on the package.

- Line your large baking pan with foil. Then place chopped vegetables and slices of chicken on it. Pour the olive oil over veggies.

- In a small bowl, combine the garlic powder, cayenne, oregano, cumin, salt, and pepper. Cover the chicken and veggies with the prepped spice mixture and toss to coat.

• Transfer that baking pan to the oven and cook for fifteen minutes. Meanwhile prepare three containers.

• Remove your baking pan from the oven and transfer cooked vegetables to containers, so they're evenly divided. Then put the baking pan with the chicken back in the oven for another ten minutes.

• When rice and chicken are cooked, divide them between containers too. Let your prepped meals cool down before storing in your fridge.

Honey-Lime Chicken with Sweet Potatoes & Asparagus

Time: 45 mins

Number of servings: 3

Ingredients:

One pound cut into smaller strips chicken breast

Three peeled and cubed sweet potatoes

Half cup honey

Juice of one lime

Two minced garlic cloves

One bunch of asparagus, ends cut off

Three Tbsp olive oil

A pinch of cinnamon

Salt and pepper to taste

Directions:

• Preheat your oven to 400°F.

• In your small bowl, mix together the honey, juice of a lime, and one of the minced garlic cloves. Stir well to combine. Place the chicken in a plastic zip-lock bag and add the prepared marinade. Toss to coat and place in the refrigerator for forty minutes.

• Line your baking pan with foil. Then place sweet potatoes on it and drizzle with olive oil. Now sprinkle cinnamon and salt over them.

- Place this baking pan with the sweet potatoes in the middle of the oven and cook for fifteen minutes.

- Meanwhile, heat one Tbsp olive oil in the skillet over medium heat. Add the reserved garlic and cook until fragrant. Then add asparagus, season with salt and pepper, and toss. Cook for six minutes, until asparagus, is bright green, but not too crispy. Transfer the cooked asparagus to three meal containers, so it's evenly divided.

- Remove any remaining garlic from the skillet and add the reserved one Tbsp olive oil. Add chicken and cook over medium heat for four minutes per side.

- Transfer the chicken and sweet potatoes to your meal containers and let them cool down before storing in your fridge.

Time: 60 mins

Number of servings: 4

Ingredients:

Four chicken breasts, skinless and boneless

One 8-oz pack of whole grain pasta

One cup shredded mozzarella cheese

One 15-oz can of crushed tomatoes

Half cup chopped onions

Quarter cup water

Four minced garlic cloves

One Tbsp sundried tomato pesto

One Tbsp olive oil

Half tsp Italian seasoning

Half tsp red pepper flakes

A pinch of dried basil

Salt and pepper to taste

Directions:

• Cook the pasta according to the info on the package.

• Season each chicken breast with salt and pepper on both sides. Heat the olive oil in your skillet over medium-high heat. Add chicken and cook for five minutes per side, until it's completely cooked through.

• Preheat your oven using broiler setting.

• Warm your skillet, add onions, and sauté for two minutes. Then add garlic and cook for just half of minute. Now add crushed tomatoes, pesto, Italian seasoning, red pepper flakes, and basil and stir well to combine.

• Bring the sauce to a simmer. Then add a quarter cup of water. Cover the lid and cook for ten minutes over low heat. Season with salt and pepper.

• Place the chicken breasts into the sauce and use a spoon to cover them with sauce. Top each chicken breast with shredded cheese. Place under the broiler for two minutes, until cheese melts.

• Finally, assemble prepared meals in your containers. Place the pasta, add some sauce and top with chicken. Let them cool down before storing in your fridge.

Time: 100 mins

Number of servings: 4

Ingredients:

Eight chicken drumsticks

One 2-lb spaghetti squash, halved and with seeds removed

Half cup organic BBQ sauce

Two Tbsp olive oil

One tsp hot sauce

Directions:

• Preheat your oven to 400°F.

• Line your baking pan with a foil and then place halved squash cut-side down. Transfer the squash to the oven and cook for twenty minutes.

• When cooked, use a fork to pull the squash flesh and shred it into strands.

• Now coat your baking dish with oil. Put cooked spaghetti squash in the bottom of dish and top with chicken. Transfer the dish to oven and bake for thirty minutes.

• Meanwhile, in a small bowl, mix together BBQ sauce and hot sauce.

• Remove the dish from the oven and coat the chicken with spicy BBQ sauce. Then bake for another thirty minutes, coating drumsticks with sauce every ten minutes.

•   Transfer the spaghetti squash to your meal containers, evenly dividing. Top with chicken and let cool down before storing in your fridge.

Time: 70 mins

Number of servings: 4

Ingredients:

One pound chicken breast, cooked and shredded

Three cups diced cauliflower

Half cup buffalo sauce

Half cup egg whites

Two chopped carrots

One diced onion

One minced garlic clove

One Tbsp olive oil

Chives for garnish

Salt and pepper to taste

Directions:

- Preheat your oven to 400°F.

- Heat the olive oil in your skillet over medium-high heat. Add onions, carrots, and garlic and sauté for three minutes, until onion is translucent.

- In a bowl, mix together chicken, cauliflower, sautéed vegetables, egg whites and buffalo sauce. Stir well to combine.

•   Line your baking pan with a parchment paper and add the prepared mixture. Cover pan with the lid and bake for twenty minutes. Then remove a cover and cook for additional thirty minutes.

•   Divide prepared casserole between your meal containers. Top with chives and let cool down before storing in your fridge.

Time: 40 mins

Number of servings: 4

Ingredients:

One pound chicken breast, cut into halves lengthwise

Two cups broccoli florets, steamed

One cup diced mozzarella cheese

Half cup pizza sauce

Half cup sliced pepperoni

One Tbsp pizza seasoning

Directions:

- Preheat your oven to 375°F.

- Place chicken on a baking pan, cover with pizza sauce and top with pizza seasoning. Bake for ten minutes.

- Now Remove the baking pan from the oven and top the chicken with mozzarella cheese. Then bake for five minutes more.

- Again remove the baking dish from the oven and add pepperoni. Return to the oven and bake for an additional fifteen minutes.

- Divide prepared chicken pizza between your meal containers. Add broccoli and let cool down before storing in your fridge.

Chicken Enchilada Bowl

Time: 40 mins

Number of servings: 6

Ingredients:

Three quartered chicken breasts

One 12-oz pack of cauliflower rice

One cup enchilada sauce

Two chopped onions

Two chopped jalapeno

One 4-oz can of green chiles

Two Tbsp olive oil

Salt and pepper to taste

Directions:

• Cook the cauliflower rice according to the info on the package.

• Heat the olive oil in a skillet over medium-high heat. Add chicken and cook for three minutes per side, until lightly brown.

• Add enchilada sauce, onions, chiles, and reduce heat to simmer. Cover the lid and cook for ten minutes.

• Now remove the chicken to a platter and shred it with two forks. Return the pulled meat to the sauce and cook uncovered for additional ten minutes.

- Divide cooked rice into meal prep containers. Top with chicken, jalapenos, and sauce. Season with salt, pepper, and let cool down before storing in your fridge.

Time: 45 mins

Number of servings: 4

Ingredients:

One and a half pounds chicken breast

One 8-oz pack of button mushrooms, sliced

One cup whole wheat couscous

One cup chicken stock

Half cup sour cream

Two minced garlic cloves

One 4-oz pack of arugula

Juice of one lemon

Three Tbsp olive oil

One tsp Dijon mustard

Salt and pepper to taste

Directions:

• Preheat your oven to 350°F and line your baking pan with parchment paper.

• In a medium pan, bring water to a boil, add couscous and cook for ten minutes. Drain and set aside.

• Heat two Tbsp olive oil in a skillet over medium heat. Season each chicken breast on all sides with salt and pepper and cook for three minutes per side, until lightly brown.

Transfer the chicken to a baking pan and bake for ten minutes.

•   In the same skillet, heat one Tbsp olive oil and over medium heat. Add garlic and cook for just half of minute. Then add mushrooms and sauté for three minutes, until browned.

•   Add chicken stock and simmer for three minutes, until reduced by half. Remove from heat and add sour cream and Dijon mustard. Stir well to combine and season with salt and pepper.

•   In a medium bowl, toss arugula with lemon juice and one Tbsp olive oil. Season with salt and pepper too.

•   Slice chicken and divide it into meal prep containers. Add couscous, arugula salad, and let cool down before storing in your fridge.

Time: 35 mins

Number of servings: 4

Ingredients:

One pound chicken breast, sliced into thick strips

One pound steamed green beans

One cup chopped tomatoes

Half cup plain bread crumbs

Quarter cup grated Parmesan cheese

Two minced garlic cloves

Five Tbsp olive oil

One tsp dried basil

Half tsp oregano

A pinch of rosemary

Salt and pepper to taste

Directions:

•	Preheat your oven to 400°F and line a large rimmed baking sheet with parchment paper.

•	In a shallow bowl, whisk together Parmesan, bread crumbs, basil, oregano, rosemary, salt, and pepper.

•	Pour olive oil in a separate shallow bowl and stir in garlic.

•	Dredge each chicken tender in olive oil and immediately coat with bread crumb mixture. Place them in a row along one side of your baking sheet.

•	Toss green beans with one Tbsp olive oil on the other side of baking sheet. Season with salt and pepper.

•	Place the baking sheet in the oven and bake for fifteen minutes. Then toss the green beans and cook for additional ten minutes.

•	Divide chicken and veggies into meal prep containers. Add tomatoes and let cool down before storing in your fridge.

Time: 40 mins

Number of servings: 4

Ingredients:

One and a half pounds skinless and boneless chicken breast, cubed

Four zucchini

Four minced garlic cloves

One cup sour cream

Quarter cup water

One Tbsp avocado oil

Salt and pepper to taste

Directions:

•   Make noodles from zucchini using your spiralizer. Divide zoodles between your meal prep containers.

•   Warm the avocado oil in a skillet over medium heat. Then add the chicken and cook for five minutes per side.

•   In a saucepan, add sour cream and cook for three minutes over low heat. Then add garlic, stir, and cook for additional three minutes. Now add water, season with salt and pepper and cook for five minutes.

•   Add chicken and prepared sauce in the meal prep containers and let cool down before storing in your fridge.

Time: 40 mins

Number of servings: 6

Ingredients:

One and a half pounds chicken breast

One pound asparagus, ends cut off

One cup brown rice

Two minced garlic cloves

Quarter cup oyster sauce

One Tbsp olive oil

Directions:

•   Preheat your oven to 400°F and line a baking sheet with foil. Cover with the oil.

•   Cook the brown rice according to the info on the package.

•   Meanwhile, in a small bowl, mix together oyster sauce and garlic.

•   Place chicken and asparagus on the baking sheet and drizzle with the prepared garlic mixture.

•   Put the baking sheet in the oven and bake for twenty minutes, until chicken is cooked through.

•   Divide cooked brown rice into meal prep containers. Top with chicken and asparagus, and let cool down before storing in your fridge.

Time: 45 mins

Number of servings: 8

Ingredients:

Two pounds skinless and boneless chicken breast, cut into bite-sized pieces

Two cups whole grain couscous

Three carrots, grated

Two and a half cups of light coconut milk

Two cups water

Half cup raisins

Half cup chopped cilantro

Two Tbsp curry powder

Two Tbsp flour

One Tbsp coconut oil

One tsp salt

Directions:

•   In a medium saucepan, mix together half cup coconut milk and water. Bring the mixture to a boil over medium-high heat and stir in couscous gradually. Remove from the stove, cover, and let sit for five minutes. Then open the lid and fluff it gently with a fork.

•   Place the chicken in a zip-lock plastic bag. Add curry powder, flour, and salt. Seal the bag and toss to coat.

•   Warm the coconut oil in a large skillet over medium heat. Add chicken and cook for five minutes, stirring frequently.

•   Now add carrots, raisins, and reserved two cups coconut milk. Bring the mixture to a boil and then reduce the heat to low. Simmer, stirring occasionally, for ten minutes.

•   Divide cooked couscous into meal prep containers. Add curried chicken and top with cilantro. Let cool down before storing in your fridge.

Time: 40 mins

Number of servings: 4

Ingredients:

Three cups cooked and shredded chicken breast

Four cups shredded cabbage

One chipotle pepper in adobo sauce, sliced

Two Tbsp adobo sauce (you have some in the same can with chipotle pepper)

One diced onion

One minced garlic clove

Half cup BBQ sauce

Half cup of apple cider vinegar

Two Tbsp olive oil mayonnaise

Two Tbsp chopped cilantro

One tsp olive oil

One tsp honey

Half celery seeds

Directions:

• In a large bowl, mix together mayonnaise, quarter cup vinegar, cilantro, celery seeds, and honey. Add cabbage, stir well to combine and refrigerate for twenty minutes.

•	Warm the olive oil in your skillet over medium-high heat. Add onions and cook for five minutes. Then add garlic and cook for just one minute.

•	Now add BBQ sauce, reserved quarter cup vinegar, chipotle pepper, and adobo sauce. Cook, stirring occasionally, for eight minutes.

•	Finally, add shredded chicken and cook, stirring frequently, for five minutes.

•	Add chicken and veggies to the meal prep containers and let cool down before storing in your fridge.

Time: 60 mins

Number of servings: 4

Ingredients:

One pound skinless and boneless chicken breast, cubed

Two cup rotini pasta, uncooked

One 8-oz pack baby bella mushrooms, sliced

Three sun-dried tomatoes, chopped

One cup shredded mozzarella

One cup milk

One cup chicken stock

Two cups chopped Tuscan kale

Two Tbsp flour

One Tbsp olive oil

Salt and pepper to taste

Directions:

- Preheat your oven to 400°F.

- In a baking pan, mix together the flour, salt, pepper, chicken stock, and milk. Then add pasta, dried tomatoes, and stir well to combine.

- Now add chicken and mushrooms, and cover the pan with a foil. Place the baking pan in the oven and bake for thirty minutes.

•	Remove the baking pan from the oven and stir everything up. Then return uncovered pan to the oven and bake for fifteen minutes more.

•	Again remove the baking pan from the oven and stir in the cheese and kale. Return to the oven and cook for another five minutes.

•	Divide cooked chicken pasta bake into meal prep containers and let cool down before storing in your fridge.

Time: 40 mins

Number of servings: 4

Ingredients:

One pound chicken breast

One cup pearl couscous

Four cups cauliflower florets

One cup chopped green beans

Half onion, chopped

Juice of half a lemon

Two Tbsp olive oil

Two Tbsp Moroccan seasoning

Salt to taste

Directions:

•   Cook the pearl couscous according to the info on the package. Stir in the lemon juice, season with salt and allow to cool.

•   Preheat your oven to 425°F.

•   Place chicken in a baking dish, sprinkle with olive oil and season with salt and Moroccan seasoning. Now put the baking dish in the oven and bake for twenty minutes, flipping once halfway. Then remove and set aside.

•   Now place cauliflower florets on the separate baking sheet. Drizzle with olive oil and season with Moroccan seasoning. Put in the oven and bake for fifteen minutes.

•   Remove the baking sheet with cauliflower from the oven and add green beans with onions. Then return uncovered pan to the oven and bake for ten minutes more.

•   Slice the chicken into strips and divide it into meal prep containers. Add couscous, veggies, and let cool down before storing in your fridge.

Time: 60 mins

Number of servings: 4

Ingredients:

Four chicken thighs, skin-on, and bone-in

One pound baby potatoes, halved

Sixteen Brussels sprouts, chopped in half

Half butternut squash, peeled and sliced

Four peeled and chopped carrots

Quarter cup melted butter

Two Tbsp white Miso paste

Two Tbsp olive oil

Two Tbsp honey

One tsp sesame oil

Salt and pepper to taste

Directions:

- Preheat your oven to 425°F.

- In a large bowl, add Brussels sprouts, potatoes, carrots, and butternut squash. Toss with olive oil, salt, and pepper.

- Transfer veggies to a large baking dish. Top with chicken thighs. Sprinkle chicken with oil, and season with salt and pepper. Place the baking dish in the oven and roast for fifty minutes, until chicken is golden.

•   Meanwhile, in a small bowl, mix together butter, miso, honey, sesame oil, and pepper. Stir well to combine and set aside.

•   Divide cooked chicken and veggies into meal prep containers and let cool down before storing in your fridge. Use 3-oz mini containers for miso butter.

Time: 50 mins

Number of servings: 4

Ingredients:

One pound skinless and boneless chicken breast, cut into 1-inch pieces

Two cups cooked brown rice

One cup diced baby bella mushrooms

One cup broccoli florets

Two diced bell peppers

One diced zucchini

Three chopped garlic cloves

Half cup soy sauce

Quarter cup honey

Four Tbsp olive oil

Two Tbsp vinegar

One Tbsp grated ginger

One Tbsp cornstarch

One Tbsp sesame seeds

One tsp garlic paste

One tsp chili flakes

Salt and pepper to taste

Directions:

•	Preheat your oven to 425°F and line a baking sheet with parchment paper.

•	Toss the mushrooms, broccoli, bell peppers, zucchini in olive oil and season with salt and pepper. Place all veggies on a baking sheet and roast for twenty minutes.

•	Cover chicken pieces with garlic paste and set aside for fifteen minutes.

•	Meanwhile, in a bowl, mix together ginger, garlic, honey, chili flakes, cornstarch, vinegar, and soy sauce. Add one and a half cups water and stir well to combine.

•	Heat one Tbsp olive oil in a pan over medium-high heat. Add the marinated chicken and cook for five minutes per side.

•	Add prepared sauce and bring to a boil, stirring continuously. Then reduce the heat to low and cook for three minutes.

•	Divide cooked rice, roast veggies, and teriyaki chicken into meal prep containers and sprinkle with sesame seeds. Let cool down before storing in your fridge.

Time: 60 mins

Number of servings: 6

Ingredients:

Two pounds skinless and boneless chicken breast, cut into 1-inch pieces

Four cups cooked quinoa

Two sweet potatoes, cut into matchsticks

One bunch asparagus, ends cut off

Four minced garlic cloves

Half cup pitted olives

Juice of two lemons

Five Tbsp olive oil

One Tbsp honey

Two tsp paprika

Two tsp cumin

Salt and pepper to taste

Directions:

• Preheat your oven to 425°F and line a baking sheet with parchment paper.

• Put chicken in a large zip-lock plastic bag. Add the honey, lemon juice, two Tbsp olive oil, garlic, paprika, cumin, salt, and pepper. Toss to coat and let chill for at least thirty minutes.

• Place the sweet potatoes on the baking sheet and toss with two Tbsp olive oil, salt, and pepper. Transfer to the oven and bake for forty minutes, flipping once halfway through cooking.

• Place the asparagus on the baking sheet and toss with the reserved one Tbsp olive oil, salt, and pepper. Transfer to the oven and cook for fifteen minutes.

• Now place the marinated chicken on the baking sheet and bake for twenty minutes.

• Divide cooked quinoa between your meal prep containers. Add chicken, sweet potatoes, asparagus, and olives. Let cool down before storing in your fridge.

Time: 40 mins

Number of servings: 4

Ingredients:

One pound skinless and boneless chicken breast, cut into 4-oz portions

Two cups cooked quinoa

One cup Greek yogurt

Two diced tomatoes

Two diced cucumber

Half onion, diced

Half cup pitted and chopped black olives

Juice of one lemon

Two Tbsp olive oil

One Tbsp red wine vinegar

One Tbsp Italian seasoning

One tsp garlic powder

Half tsp cornstarch

Half tsp onion powder

Half tsp paprika

Salt and pepper to taste

Directions:

•   Preheat your oven to 450°F and line a baking sheet with a foil.

•   In a small bowl, mix together Italian seasoning, garlic powder, cornstarch, onion powder, paprika, salt, and pepper.

•   Place the chicken on the baking sheet and coat evenly with the mix seasoning. Transfer to the oven and bake for twenty minutes.

•   Meanwhile, in a large bowl, mix together cucumber, tomatoes, onion and olives. Add one Tbsp olive oil, lemon juice, vinegar and stir well to combine.

•   Divide cooked chicken, quinoa, and Greek salad between your meal prep containers. Let cool down before storing in your fridge.

Easy Jerk Chicken

Time: 30 mins

Number of servings: 4

Ingredients:

One pound chicken breast, cut into 1-inch pieces

Two cups cooked yellow rice

One 15-oz can of black beans, drained and rinsed

Two cups diced pineapple

Half cup diced onion

Quarter cup chopped cilantro

One Tbsp olive oil

One Tbsp Jamaican Jerk Seasoning

Directions:

• In the medium bowl, mix together pineapple, onion, and cilantro. Stir to combine and set aside.

• Sprinkle the chicken pieces with Jamaican jerk seasoning and stir to coat.

• Heat olive oil in a skillet over medium heat. Add chicken and cook for three minutes per side, until cooked through.

• Divide cooked rice, black beans, chicken, and prepared pineapple salsa between your meal prep containers. Let cool down before storing in your fridge.

Time: 45 mins

Number of servings: 4

Ingredients:

One pound ground chicken

Three cups whole grain pasta

Two cups butternut squash, cubed

One 4-oz package of goat cheese

Quarter cup chopped walnuts

Two minced garlic cloves

Three Tbsp olive oil

Two Tbsp balsamic vinegar

Chopped basil for garnish

Salt and pepper to taste

Directions:

• Preheat your oven to 400°F and line a baking sheet with a parchment paper.

• Toss the butternut squash with two Tbsp olive oil and place on the lined baking sheet. Season with salt and pepper and bake for thirty minutes.

• Meanwhile, cook the whole grain pasta according to the info on the package and set aside.

- Heat the remaining one Tbsp olive oil in a skillet over medium heat. Add garlic and cook for a minute. Then add ground chicken and cook for five minutes, stirring frequently.

- Reduce heat to low and add in walnuts and balsamic vinegar. Cook for three minutes and remove from the heat.

- Divide cooked pasta between meal prep containers. Top with the chicken mixture, butternut squash, goat cheese, and chopped basil. Let cool down before storing in your fridge.

Italian Chicken Bowls

Time: 30 mins

Number of servings: 4

Ingredients:

Two pounds chicken breast, cut into bite-sized pieces

Two cups broccoli florets

One cup diced tomatoes

One chopped zucchini

One chopped onion

Four minced garlic cloves

Two Tbsp olive oil

Two tsp dried basil

Two tsp marjoram

Two tsp rosemary

Two tsp thyme

One tsp paprika

Salt and pepper to taste

Directions:

• Preheat your oven to 400°F and line a baking sheet with a foil.

• In a small bowl, mix together basil, marjoram, rosemary, thyme, paprika, salt, and pepper.

•   Place the chicken and vegetables on the baking sheet and sprinkle with the garlic and mixed spices. Then drizzle with olive oil and transfer to the oven. Bake for twenty minutes.

•   Divide cooked chicken and veggies between meal prep containers, and let cool down before storing in your fridge.

Chicken in Peanut Lemon Sauce

Time: 65 mins

Number of servings: 4

Ingredients:

One pound chicken skinless and boneless breast

One cup brown rice

Three cups diced broccoli

Three cups diced carrots

One cup chicken stock

One cup water

Quarter cup creamy peanut butter

Two Tbsp olive oil

One Tbsp lemon zest

One Tbsp soy sauce

One Tbsp rice vinegar

One Tbsp lemon juice

Half Tbsp brown sugar

Half tsp sesame oil

Salt to taste

Directions:

- Cook the brown rice according to the info on the package, adding the salt, chicken stock and lemon zest to the cooking water.

- Preheat your oven to 425°F and line a baking sheet with parchment paper.

- Toss the broccoli and carrots with one Tbsp olive oil and place on the baking sheet.

- Place the chicken in a small baking pan and cover with one Tbsp olive oil and soy sauce.

- Transfer the chicken and veggies to the oven. Bake for twenty minutes, flipping chicken and stirring veggies once halfway through cooking.

- Meanwhile, gently heat the peanut butter in a microwave-safe dish. Then stir in lemon juice, sesame oil, rice vinegar, and brow sugar.

- Slice cooked chicken. Divide cooked brown rice between meal prep containers and top with sliced chicken and vegetables. Drizzle with prepared peanut lemon sauce and let cool down before storing in your fridge.

Time: 70 mins

Number of servings: 4

Ingredients:

One pound lean ground turkey

One cup brown rice

One 12-oz can of whole kernel corn

Two cups diced tomatoes

Quarter cup shredded mozzarella cheese

One minced onion

One minced jalapeno

Zest of one lime

Juice of half a lime

Two Tbsp olive oil

Two Tbsp taco seasoning mix

Salt to taste

Directions:

•   Cook brown rice according to the info on the package, adding the salt and lime zest to the cooking water.

•   Heat olive oil in a skillet over medium high heat. Add ground turkey and cook for ten minutes, breaking it apart with a spatula.

•   In a large bowl, mix together tomatoes, jalapeno, onions, and lime juice. Season with salt and stir well to combine.

•   Divide cooked brown rice into your meal prep containers. Then add cooked taco meat, prepared salsa, and corn kernels. Let cool down before storing in your fridge.

Time: 35 mins

Number of servings: 4

Ingredients:

One pound ground turkey

Four cups cauliflower rice

One cup baby spinach

Half cup chopped basil

One bunch bok choy, chopped

Two sliced bell peppers

One diced onion

Half cup coconut aminos

Three Tbsp olive oil

Two tsp minced fresh ginger

Two tsp chili paste

One tsp fish sauce

Salt and pepper to taste

Directions:

• Heat two Tbsp olive oil in a skillet over medium high heat. Add ground turkey, two Tbsp coconut aminos, one tsp chili paste, one tsp ginger, half tsp fish sauce. Stir and cook for five minutes.

- Then add chopped basil, season with salt and pepper and cook for additional five minutes. Transfer cooked turkey to a platter and set aside.

- Add one Tbsp olive oil, onions, and bell peppers in a skillet. Cook for three minutes over medium heat, until onion is translucent. Add bok choy, spinach, and cook for five minutes, until softened. Then transfer veggies to a platter and set aside.

- Pour the remaining one Tbsp olive oil in a skillet. Then add cauliflower rice, season with salt and pepper, and cook for five minutes, stirring occasionally.

- In a small saucepan, combine the remaining coconut aminos, minced ginger, chili paste, and fish sauce.

- Now divide cooked turkey, veggies, and cauliflower rice between your meal prep containers. Then top with the prepared sauce and let cool down before storing in your fridge.

Time: 45 mins

Number of servings: 4

Ingredients:

One pound ground turkey breast

Two chopped sweet potatoes

One cup chopped green onions

Two sliced tomatoes

Half of onion, sliced

Eight lettuce leaves

Two Tbsp coconut oil

One Tbsp olive oil

One tsp cumin

A pinch of cayenne pepper

Salt and pepper

Directions:

- Preheat your oven to 400°F.

- In your bowl, mix together olive oil, cayenne, salt, and pepper. Add sweet potatoes and toss to coat.

- Line your baking pan with foil. Then place sweet potatoes on it and bake for thirty minutes, flipping once halfway.

- Meanwhile, in a large bowl, mix together ground turkey, green onions, cumin, salt, and pepper. Stir well to combine and form eight patties with your hands.

- Heat the coconut oil in your skillet over medium-high heat. Add patties and cook for eight minutes per side.

- Now assemble prepared meals in your containers. Place the patties on a lettuce leave, add onions and tomatoes. Then add baked sweet potatoes. Let them cool down before storing in your fridge.

Time: 70 mins

Number of servings: 8

Ingredients:

Two pounds turkey breast, skin-on and bone-in

Two bunches chopped Swiss chard

Two sliced carrots

One bunch chopped spinach

One sliced bell pepper

One sliced onion

Three minced garlic clove

Juice of half a lemon

One Tbsp olive oil

One Tbsp chopped chives

One Tbsp chopped parsley

One Tbsp chopped thyme

Salt and pepper to taste

Directions:

- Preheat your oven to 350°F.

- Disperse one sliced carrot, half of sliced onion, and two minced garlic cloves along the bottom of a baking dish.

- In a small bowl, mix together thyme, parsley, and chives. Staff the mixture under the skin of the turkey breast. Season meat with salt and pepper.

- Place the turkey breast in the baking dish, on top of the veggies. Then pour ¼-inch of water in the dish, place it in the oven, and bake for forty minutes.

- Meanwhile, warm the olive oil in your skillet over medium heat. Add bell pepper and the remaining carrot, onion, garlic. Sauté for five minutes and then add a half of Swiss chard and cook until it's wilted. Repeat with remaining chard and spinach, one by one.

- Now slice the cooked turkey and divide between your meal prep containers. Add vegetables from the skillet and let cool down before storing in your fridge.

Eggs are very popular in meal plans for both losing weight and building muscle. Due to their protein power, eggs can help to be more satisfied during weight loss process. And several studies show that egg-eaters achieve a greater reduction in waistline, compared to a control group. Moreover, an egg is a budget-friendly, easy, and versatile food.

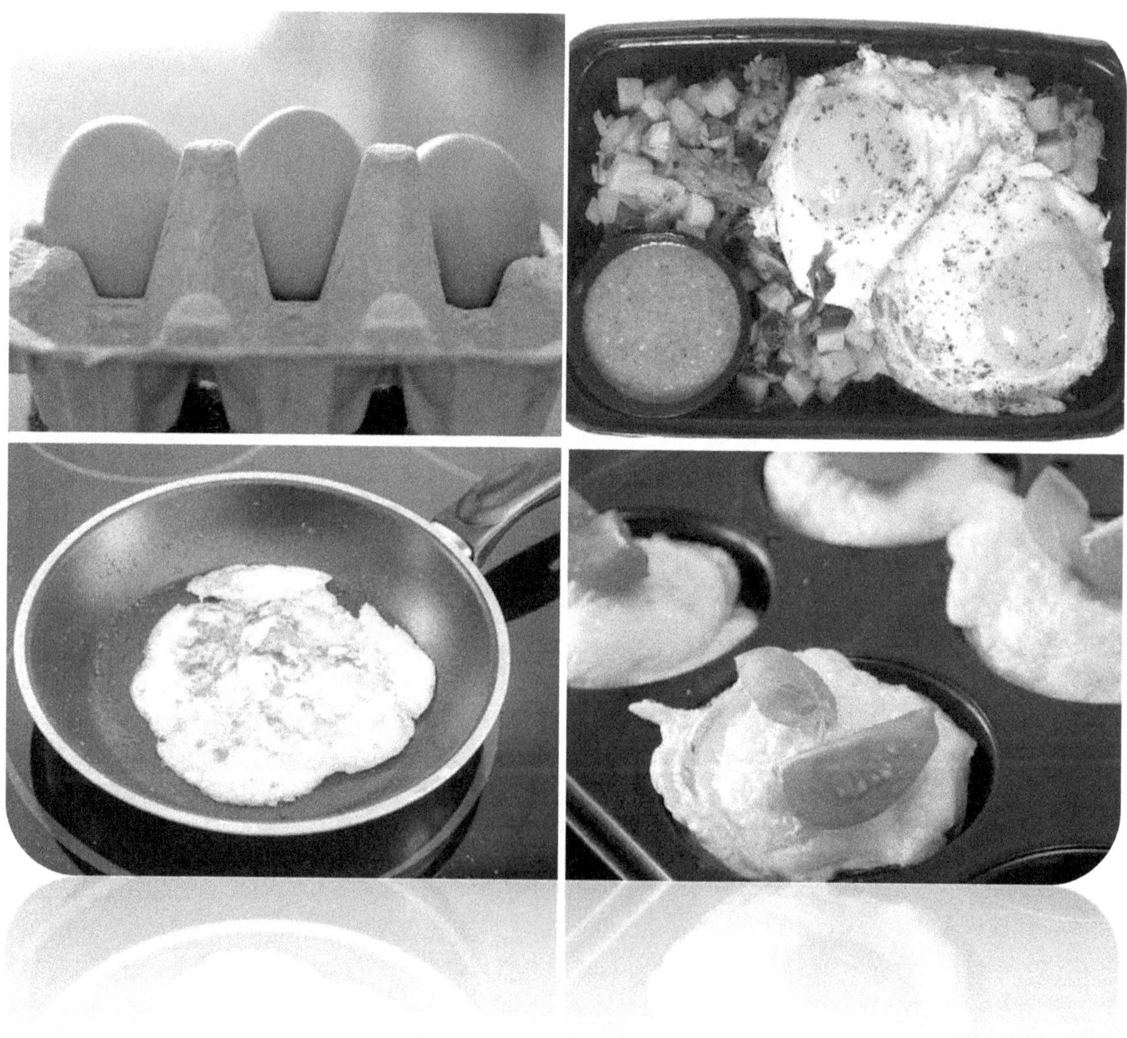

One large chicken egg has just 70 calories and provides you with 18 vitamins and minerals, and most of these essential nutrients reside in the yolk. That's why consuming whole eggs results in significantly greater muscle growth versus eating egg whites only.

One large egg satisfies about ¼ of your daily needs for choline, biotin, and selenium. Choline is a nutrient that's important for brain health, nerve function, muscle movement, and maintaining energy levels. There is some evidence that many people do not get enough choline in their diets. That's why eggs are sometimes called "brain food" - since they supply high amounts of choline.

Time: 10 mins

Number of servings: 4

Ingredients:

Eight eggs

Eight small organic sausages, cooked

Two cups broccoli florets, steamed

Quarter cup of milk

Two Tbsp olive oil

One Tbsp dried turmeric

One tsp dried parsley

Salt and pepper to taste

Directions:

•	In your large bowl, whisk together the milk, eggs, turmeric, parsley, salt, and pepper.

•	Heat the olive oil in a skillet over medium heat. Add the prepared mixture and cook for five minutes, stirring constantly.

•	Transfer the eggs to your meal containers, evenly dividing. Add sausages, steamed broccoli and let cool down before storing in your fridge.

Sausage Hash Brown Casserole

Time: 60 mins

Number of servings: 6

Ingredients:

Six eggs

Six sausages, pre-cooked

Four cups shredded potatoes

One and a half cup egg whites

One cup spinach

One Tbsp olive oil

Salt and pepper to taste

Directions:

- Preheat your oven to 350°F.

- In your large bowl, whisk together egg whites and eggs. Then add shredded potatoes, sausages, spinach and stir well to combine.

- Coat your baking dish with the olive oil. Pour in the prepared mixture and bake for fifty minutes.

- Transfer the casserole to your meal containers, evenly dividing. Let it cool down before storing in your fridge.

Time: 40 mins

Number of servings: 6

Ingredients:

Eight eggs

One chopped bell pepper

Half onion, chopped

Half zucchini, shredded

Two minced garlic cloves

Two cups chopped arugula

Quarter cup shredded Parmesan cheese

One Tbsp olive oil

Salt and pepper to taste

Directions:

•   Preheat your oven to 375°F and coat a muffin tin with cooking spray.

•   Heat the olive oil in a skillet over medium heat. Add onion, garlic, and sauté for four minutes. Then add zucchini, bell pepper, and cook for two minutes more.

•   In a large bowl, whisk together eggs, cheese, arugula, salt and pepper.

•   Now place sautéed veggies at the bottom of each muffin tin. Then fill each muffin tin evenly with prepared egg mixture. Place in the oven and bake for twenty minutes.

•   Transfer egg muffins to your meal containers and let them cool down before storing in your fridge.

Time: 40 mins

Number of servings: 8

Ingredients:

Twelve eggs

Two cups sliced bell peppers

One cup sliced organic sausage

One cup shredded cheese

Half cup heavy cream

One Tbsp olive oil

Salt and pepper to taste

Directions:

• Preheat your oven to 350°F.

• In your large bowl, whisk together eggs, heavy cream, salt, and pepper.

• Heat the olive oil in a skillet over medium heat. Then add sausage and cook for five minutes, until brown. Transfer sausage to a platter and set aside.

• Add prepared egg mixture to skillet and cook for five minutes. Then place the skillet in the oven and bake for twenty minutes.

• Remove from the oven and add sausage, peppers, and cheese. Return to the oven and broil for three minutes and then let sit for five minutes.

- • Slice the cooked pizza and divide between your meal prep containers. As always, let cool down before storing in your fridge.

Time: 40 mins

Number of servings: 8

Ingredients:

Four large bell peppers, seeded and halved lengthwise

Nine eggs

Half cup black beans

Half cup cooked quinoa

Half cup boiled potatoes, chopped

Half cup shredded cheese

Half cup chopped spinach

Salt and pepper to taste

Directions:

• Preheat your oven to 400°F.

• Place the peppers on a baking sheet and cook for five minutes.

• In a large bowl, whisk together eggs, black beans, quinoa, potatoes, and spinach. Stir well to combine, and season with salt and pepper.

• Spoon the prepared egg mixture into each pepper, and top with the shredded cheese. Now place back the baking sheet in the oven and bake for twenty minutes.

- Divide cooked bell peppers between your meal prep containers, and let cool down before storing in your fridge.

Seafood provides you with high amounts of protein that tastes good. It also has low levels of saturated fat and contains vitamin E. Furthermore, fatty fish, like salmon, tuna, trout, are packed with Omega-3 fatty acids.

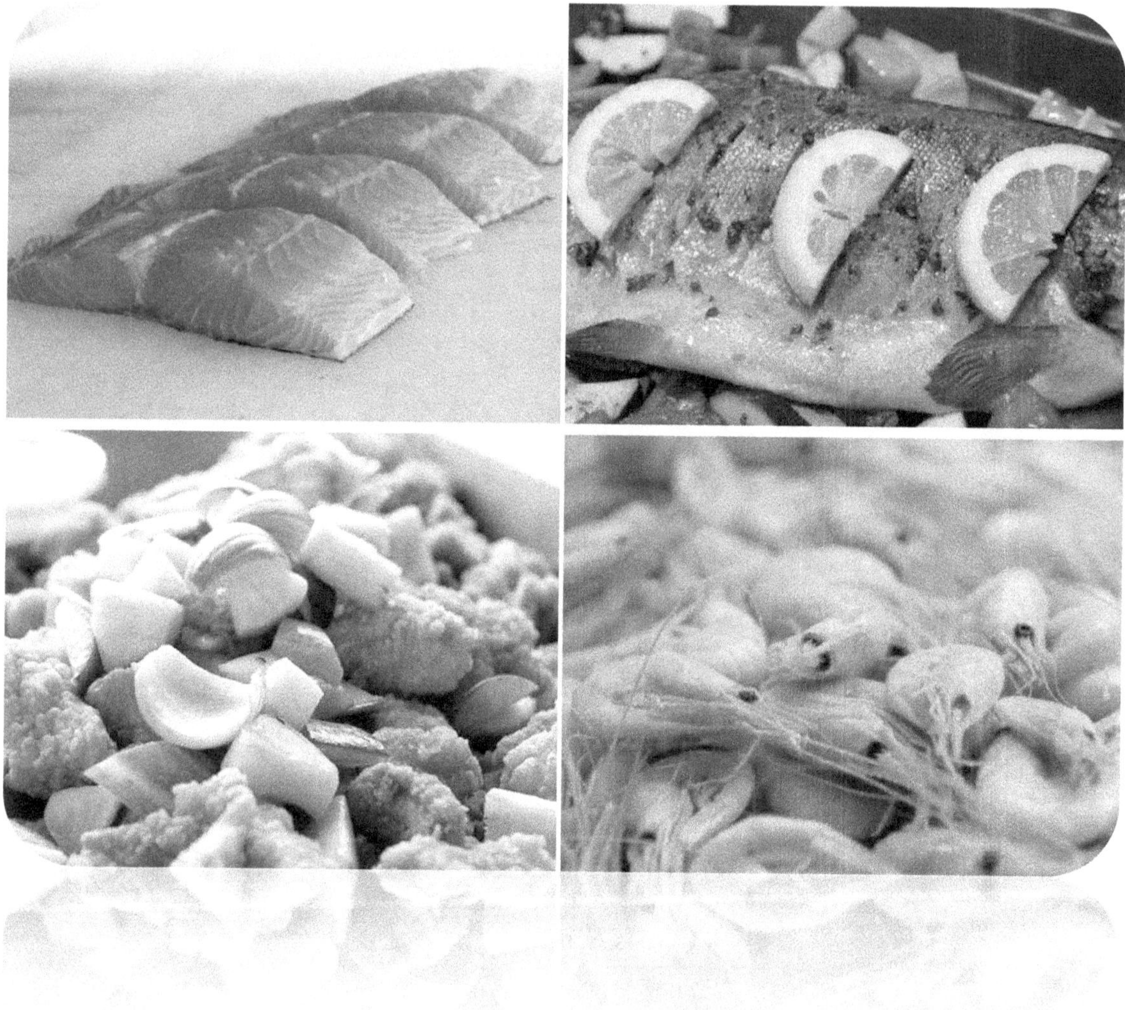

These beneficial fats can reduce the risk of heart attacks, strokes, and arrhythmias. According to statistics, regular fish consumption reduces the risk of heart attack by 40%.

Also, consuming Omega-3 can improve brain health and lower the risk of developing Alzheimer's disease. Consuming more seafood helps us have a more positive outlook on life and even has potential to treat depression.

There is a wide variety of fish and seafood to choose from. Mercury content is a serious concern with seafood. Mostly, the fish highest in healthy Omega-3 fatty acids are the lowest in mercury.

Time: 50 mins

Number of servings: 3

Ingredients:

One 12-oz pack of salmon fillets

Two sweet potatoes, peeled and cubed

Two cups broccoli florets

Two Tbsp olive oil

Two Tbsp lemon juice

One Tbsp butter, melted

Half tsp cumin powder

A pinch of garlic powder

Directions:

• Preheat your oven to 400°F

• Line the baking pan with a parchment paper and add the sweet potatoes. Drizzle with olive oil, season with cumin, salt, and pepper, and toss to coat. Put cubed sweet potatoes in the oven and set a timer for fifteen minutes.

• Meanwhile, in a small mix together melted butter, garlic powder, lemon juice, salt, and pepper. Stir well to combine.

• Line another baking pan with foil and place the salmon fillets skin-side down. Drizzle the fish with the prepared lemon-butter sauce. Now place broccoli florets on the same baking pan, drizzle them with olive oil and season with the salt and pepper.

- When the timer on the sweet potatoes goes off, remove and flip them over. Put back in the oven along with salmon and broccoli and bake for fifteen minutes.

- Divide the salmon, sweet potatoes, and broccoli into meal prep containers and let them cool down before storing in your fridge.

Salmon Fajita

Time: 30 mins

Number of servings: 4

Ingredients:

One pound salmon fillets, cut into four portions

Two sliced bell peppers

One sliced onion

Two Tbsp olive oil

Fajita seasoning to taste

Directions:

• Preheat your oven to 400°F.

• Line the baking pan with a foil and add the salmon and vegetables. Drizzle with olive oil and season with fajita seasoning.

• Place the pan with fish and veggies in the oven and bake for twenty minutes.

• Divide cooked fish and veggies into meal prep containers and let them cool down before storing in your fridge.

Time: 30 mins (and one hour for marinating)

Number of servings: 4

Ingredients:

One pound salmon fillets

One 8-oz pack baby bella mushrooms

Four halved baby bok choy, ends cut off

One green onion, sliced

Juice of half lemon

One Tbsp sesame seeds, toasted

One Tbsp coconut aminos

One Tbsp olive oil

One tsp sesame oil

One tsp grated ginger

Salt and pepper to taste

Directions:

- In a bowl, mix together olive oil, sesame oil, lemon juice, coconut aminos, ginger, salt, and pepper. Drizzle the salmon with the half of prepared marinade, cover, and place in your fridge for one hour.

- Preheat your oven to 400°F and line a baking sheet with foil.

•	Place the mushrooms and bok choy on a baking sheet and drizzle with remaining marinade.

•	Place salmon skin-side down on the same baking sheet and bake for twenty minutes.

•	Divide cooked salmon and veggies between meal prep containers and top with sesame seeds and green onions. Let cool down before storing in your fridge.

Time: 40 mins

Number of servings: 4

Ingredients:

One pound salmon fillets

Two cups diced potatoes

Two cups riced cauliflower

Two cups sliced tomatoes

Two Tbsp tamarind sauce

Three Tbsp olive oil

Directions:

• Preheat your oven to 425°F and line the baking sheet with a foil.

• Toss potatoes with olive oil and place on the baking sheet. Put in the oven and bake for fifteen minutes.

• Remove the baking sheet and place salmon, skin-side down. Return in the oven and bake for an additional ten minutes.

• Meanwhile, heat one Tbsp oil in a skillet over medium heat and add riced cauliflower. Cook, stirring frequently, for three minutes. Then remove from the heat.

• Divide cooked salmon, potatoes, and cauliflower between meal prep containers and top with tamarind sauce. Let cool down before storing in your fridge.

Time: 40 mins

Number of servings: 8

Ingredients:

Two pounds salmon fillets

Juice of half lemon

Three minced garlic cloves

Three Tbsp rice vinegar

Two Tbsp chopped basil

One Tbsp soy sauce

One Tbsp honey

One Tbsp grated ginger

Two tsp sriracha sauce

Salt to taste

Directions:

• Preheat your oven to 375°F and line the baking sheet with a foil.

• Season salmon with salt and place in the center of baking sheet.

• In your small bowl, whisk together honey, lemon juice, vinegar, ginger, garlic, sriracha, and basil. Pour prepared marinade over fish and wrap tightly in the foil.

- Bake for twenty minutes, then unwrap the foil and broil for five minutes more.

- Divide cooked salmon between meal prep containers and let cool down before storing in your fridge.

Tuna, Veggie and Quinoa Salad

Time: 10 mins

Number of servings: 3

Ingredients:

Two 5-oz cans of tuna in water

One cup quinoa

One cup plain Greek yogurt

Two Tbsp diced radish

Two Tbsp dried parsley

One tsp lemon juice

Half tsp fresh dill

Salt and pepper to taste

Six endive leaves

Directions:

•   In your large bowl, mix together all ingredients and stir well to combine.

•   Place endive leaves at the bottom of your meal prep containers. Then add prepared salad and store in your fridge.

Time: 40 mins

Number of servings: 4

Ingredients:

One pound sushi grade tuna, cubed

One avocado, cubed

Half mango, cubed

One cup brown rice

Two Tbsp coconut aminos

One tsp coconut vinegar

One tsp sesame oil

One tsp sesame seeds

One tsp maple syrup

A pinch of garlic powder

Directions:

• Cook brown rice according to the info on the package.

• Meanwhile, in a bowl, whisk together coconut aminos, maple syrup, vinegar, garlic powder, sesame oil and seeds. Then add tuna, gently stir, and marinate for at least ten minutes.

• Now add avocado and mix together.

• Divide cooked brown rice between meal prep containers and top with tuna poke and mango.

Creamy Tuna Noodle Casserole

Time: 40 mins

Number of servings: 4

Ingredients:

Two 5-oz cans of tuna in oil, drained

One 9-oz package of egg noodles

One cup frozen green peas

One cup milk

One cup chicken stock

Half cup shredded cheddar cheese

Three Tbsp melted butter

Three Tbsp all-purpose flour

Two Tbsp breadcrumbs

Two Tbsp olive oil

Salt and pepper to taste

Directions:

• Preheat your oven to 375°F and grease your baking dish.

• In a saucepan, whisk together milk, stock, butter, and flour. Cook, stirring occasionally, for ten minutes over medium heat. Season with salt and pepper.

• Bring a pot of salted water to a boil and cook egg noodles for five minutes. Then drain them and transfer to the baking dish. Add tuna, green peas, and prepared sauce. Stir well and spread evenly in the baking dish.

•	Sprinkle shredded cheese and breadcrumbs over baking dish. Then drizzle with olive oil and transfer the casserole to the oven and bake for twenty-five minutes.

•	Slice the cooked casserole, divide it between meal prep containers, and let cool down before storing in your fridge.

Time: 30 mins

Number of servings: 6

Ingredients:

Four 6-oz tilapia fillets

Two cups cooked quinoa

One 15-oz can of black beans, drained and rinsed

One 15-oz can of corn, drained

One sliced avocado

Half cup shredded cabbage

One Tbsp olive oil

One and a half tsp paprika

One tsp garlic powder

Half tsp cumin

Half tsp salt

A pinch of ground red pepper

Directions:

•　　In your small bowl, mix together the paprika, garlic powder, cumin, salt, and red pepper. Pat the fish dry and season with the prepared blend.

•　　Warm the olive oil in a skillet over medium-high heat. Add tilapia and cook for three minutes per side. Then transfer fish to a platter, let cool, and cut into 1-inch pieces.

- Divide cooked quinoa with tilapia between your meal prep containers. Then layer corn, black beans, shredded cabbage, and avocado. Let cool down before storing in your fridge.

Sheet Pan Cod with Mushrooms and Onion

Time: 40 mins

Number of servings: 4

Ingredients:

One pound cod fillets

One 14-oz package of pearl onions

One 8-oz package baby bella mushrooms, sliced

Two Tbsp dried parsley

Two tsp dried thyme

Salt and pepper to taste

Directions:

•   Preheat your oven to 375°F and line the baking pan with parchment paper.

•   Place the fish, mushrooms, and onions onto the baking pan. Sprinkle with parsley, thyme, salt, and pepper. Place the baking pan in the oven and bake for thirty minutes.

•   Divide cooked fish, mushrooms, and onions between your meal prep containers, and let cool down before storing in your fridge.

Time: 50 mins

Number of servings: 4

Ingredients:

One pound cod fillet

Two cups brown rice

Two Tbsp soy sauce

One Tbsp garlic powder

One Tbsp sugar

Two tsp sesame seeds

One tsp ground ginger

Directions:

- Cook the brown rice according to the info on the package.

- Meanwhile, preheat your oven to 375°F and line the baking pan with parchment paper.

- Place the fish onto the baking pan and drizzle with soy sauce. Then sprinkle with ginger, garlic powder, sugar, and place the baking pan in the oven. Bake for twenty minutes.

- Divide cooked brown rice and cod between your meal prep containers, and let cool down before storing in your fridge.

Time: 30 mins

Number of servings: 3

Ingredients:

Two fillets Atlantic Cod

Two cups potatoes, diced

Two cups diced tomatoes

Four Tbsp olive oil

A pinch of fresh thyme

Salt and pepper to taste

Directions:

• Preheat your oven to 400°F

• Line the baking pan with a foil and add the potatoes. Drizzle with two Tbsp olive oil, season salt, and pepper, and toss to coat. Put the pan with potatoes in the oven and set a timer for fifteen minutes.

• Remove the pan with potatoes and flip them over. Add in the cod and tomatoes. Drizzle with reserved olive oil and season with salt, pepper, and thyme. Return to the oven and bake for ten minutes.

• Divide cooked fish and veggies into meal prep containers and let them cool down before storing in your fridge.

Time: 40 mins

Number of servings: 4

Ingredients:

One pound pre-cooked shrimp, frozen

One 20-oz can of pineapple chunks, no sugar added

One Tbsp garlic powder

Half tsp black pepper

Directions:

• Preheat your oven to 375°F and line the baking pan with parchment paper.

• Place the shrimp, bell peppers, and pineapple chunks onto the baking pan. Place this baking pan in the oven and bake for thirty minutes, flipping once through the cooking.

• Divide cooked shrimp, bell peppers, and pineapples between your meal prep containers, and let cool down before storing in your fridge.

Time: 40 mins

Number of servings: 3

Ingredients:

One pound thawed frozen shrimp

Two cups chickpea pasta

One cup sliced baby bella mushrooms

Half cup Parmesan cheese, shredded

One bunch asparagus, ends cut off

One minced garlic clove

Three Tbsp butter, melted

Two Tbsp olive oil

Salt and pepper to taste

Directions:

•   Heat one Tbsp olive oil in the skillet over medium heat. Add asparagus and mushrooms and sauté for five minutes, stirring occasionally. Then transfer cooked veggies to your meal containers, evenly dividing.

•   Cook the chickpea pasta according to the info on the package.

•   Meanwhile, heat the remaining Tbsp olive oil in the skillet over medium heat. Add garlic and cook for just half of minute. Then add shrimp, season with salt and pepper, and cook for three minutes per side. Now add cooked shrimp to your meal containers in even portions.

•   Add melted butter to the cooked and drained pasta and stir well. Then add Parmesan, salt, and pepper and stir again. Finally, transfer the pasta to your meal containers, evenly dividing. Let them cool down before storing in your fridge.

Shrimp, Veggies, and Cauliflower Rice

Time: 20 mins

Number of servings: 4

Ingredients:

One pound shrimp, chopped

Two cups mixed chopped veggies

Two cups cauliflower rice

Two Tbsp olive oil

Two Tbsp soy sauce

Salt to taste

Directions:

•   Heat one Tbsp olive oil in your skillet over medium heat and add cauliflower rice. Cook, stirring frequently, for three minutes. In last minute of cooking add soy sauce. Then transfer to a bowl and set aside.

•   Add olive oil and increase heat to medium-high. Then add shrimp and cook for two minutes per side.

•   Now add chopped veggies, reduce heat to low, cover, and cook for six minutes. Remove from the heat and stir in cooked cauliflower rice.

•   Divide between meal prep containers and let cool down before storing in your fridge.

Time: 60 mins

Number of servings: 4

Ingredients:

One pound shrimp, peeled and deveined

Two cups cooked quinoa

One 15-oz can of black beans, drained and rinsed

One sliced avocado

Half cup chopped cilantro

Juice of one lime

One tsp soy sauce

One tsp BBQ seasoning

One tsp lemon pepper seasoning

Salt and pepper to taste

Directions:

•   Place the shrimp in a zip-lock bag. Add lime juice, soy sauce, lemon pepper, BBQ seasoning, and gently toss to coat. Seal the bag and place in your fridge for thirty minutes.

•   Meanwhile, add black beans to a saucepan, and cook for four minutes over medium-high heat. Then remove saucepan from the heat and set aside.

•   Place the marinated shrimp into a grill pan and cook for three minutes over medium heat, until bright pink.

- Divide cooked quinoa, shrimp, black beans, and sliced avocado between your meal prep containers. Let cool down before storing in your fridge.

Time: 40 mins

Number of servings: 4

Ingredients:

Four 6-oz halibut fillets, skinless

One pound peeled and chopped peaches

One cup chopped bell peppers

Half cup chopped arugula

Quarter cup green onions, sliced

Juice of two lemons

Half seeded and minced habanero pepper

One Tbsp chopped fresh oregano

Two minced garlic clove

Two Tbsp olive oil

One tsp paprika

Salt and pepper to taste

Directions:

•   In a shallow dish, whisk together one Tbsp lemon juice, one Tbsp olive oil, one garlic clove, and paprika. Add fish to the mixture, toss to coat, cover, and marinate for fifteen minutes.

•   Meanwhile, in your large bowl, mix together the peaches, bell pepper, habanero pepper, green onions, arugula, oregano, one minced garlic clove, salt, and pepper. Stir well to combine and place in the fridge.

•	Warm remaining olive oil in a skillet over medium-high heat. Remove the fish from marinade and cook for three minutes per side.

•	Divide cooked halibut and salsa into meal prep containers, and let cool down before storing in your fridge.

Pan-Fried Trout with Tomato Basil Sauce

Time: 30 mins

Number of servings: 4

Ingredients:

Four 6-oz trout fillets

Two cups diced tomatoes

Quarter cup chopped pancetta

Quarter cup chopped fresh basil

One minced garlic clove

One Tbsp olive oil

Four lemon wedges

Salt and pepper to taste

Directions:

•   Add pancetta in a medium skillet and cook for four minutes. Then add tomatoes, garlic, salt, pepper and cook for three minutes. Remove your skillet from the heat and stir in chopped basil.

•   Warm olive oil in a large skillet over medium-high heat. Season trout with salt and pepper, and cook for two minutes per side.

•   Divide cooked trout between your meal prep containers. Add tomato mixture and top with lemon wedges. Let cool down before storing in your fridge.

Time: 20 mins

Number of servings: 4

Ingredients:

Four 6-oz tilapia fillets

Three cups basmati rice

One cup chopped bell pepper

One cup chopped green onions

Two minced garlic cloves

One 14-oz can of light coconut milk

Two Tbsp chopped cilantro

One Tbsp brown sugar

One Tbsp soy sauce

One Tbsp olive oil

Two tsp minced ginger

Two tsp red curry paste

One tsp curry powder

One tsp toasted sesame oil

Half tsp ground cumin

Salt to taste

Four lime wedges

Directions:

- Preheat your broiler and coat a baking sheet with cooking spray.

- Warm olive oil in a skillet over medium heat. Add ginger, garlic and cook for one minute. Then add onions and pepper and cook for another one minute. Now stir in cumin, curry powder, curry paste, and cook for one minute more.

- Add coconut milk, soy sauce, brown sugar, and bring the mixture to a simmer. Then remove from heat, add cilantro and stir well to combine.

- Season the fish with salt and place on the baking sheet. Broil for seven minutes, until tilapia flakes easily when tested.

- Divide cooked fish between your meal prep containers. Add prepared coconut-curry sauce and top with lime wedges. Let cool down before storing in your fridge.

Time: 60 mins

Number of servings: 4

Ingredients:

One pound tilapia fillets, cut into six pieces

One cup breadcrumbs

Two minced garlic cloves

Two Tbsp melted butter

Salt and pepper to taste

Lemon wedges for garnish

Directions:

•   Preheat your oven to 400°F and line the baking pan with parchment paper.

•   In a small bowl, mix together breadcrumbs, garlic, butter, salt, and pepper. Coat the fish pieces with the prepared mixture evenly.

•   Place tilapia on the baking sheet and bake for twenty minutes, until golden brown.

•   Divide cooked fish between your meal prep containers. Add a side dish and vegetables of choice, and let cool down before storing in your fridge.

Red meat contains huge amounts of protein, B vitamins, vitamin D, selenium, and zinc. And half of the fats found in beef are heart-healthy monounsaturated fats. However, conventional beef has a different saturated fat profile than grass fed beef.

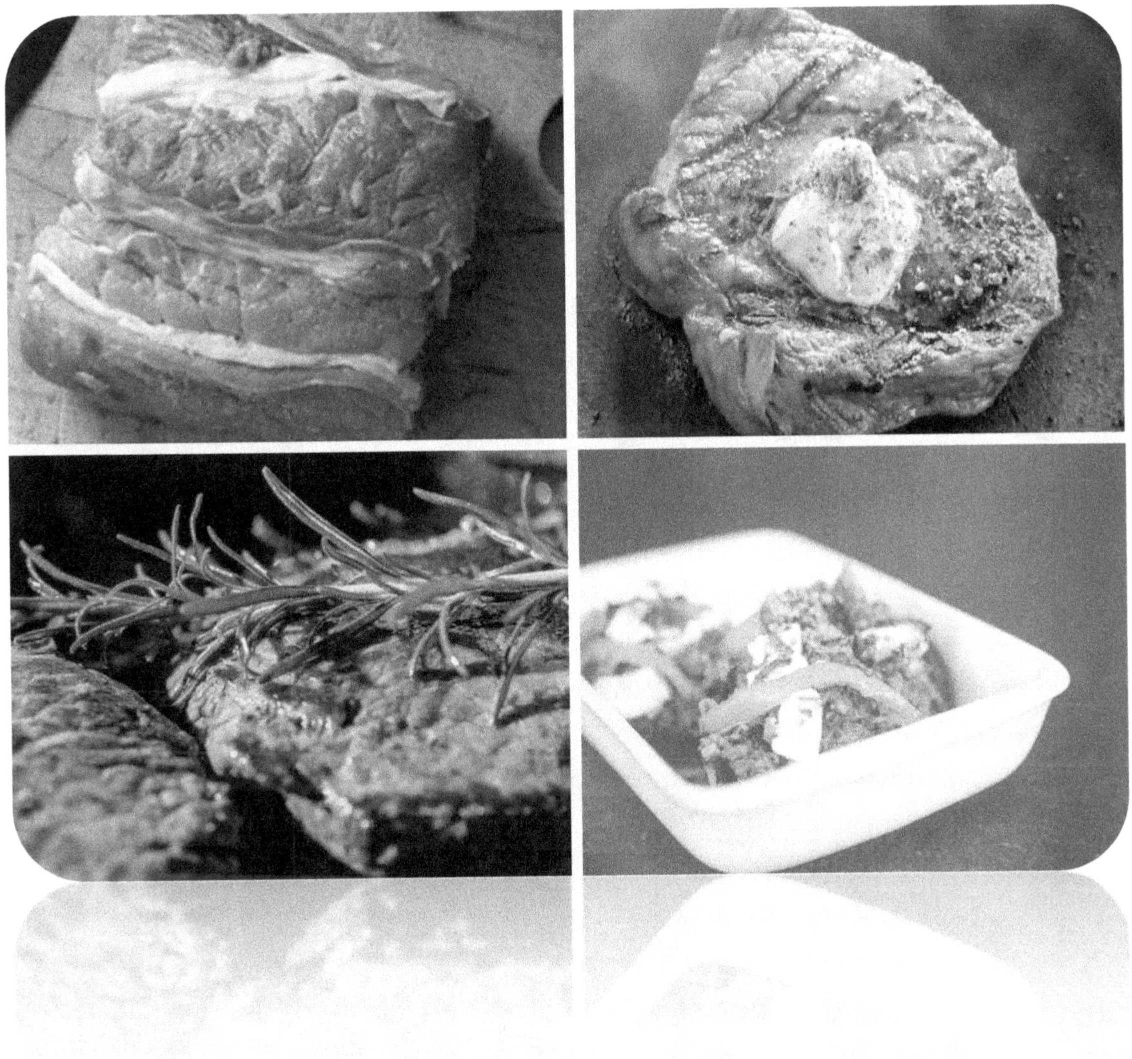

There is some evidence that many people are deficient in iron. Beef contains heme-iron - the more bio-available form of iron, which works much more efficiently than iron from veggies. Moreover, red meat has the highest rate of iron over other usually consumed meats such as poultry and pork.

Still, it is essential to limit the amount of beef you are consuming. Consider swapping some of your animal-based proteins for plant-based alternatives. Plan a couple of 'meatless' days each week.

Time: 60 mins

Number of servings: 6

Ingredients:

Two and a half pounds eye round roast

One pound Brussels sprouts, halved

Two chopped potatoes

One chopped onion

Three Tbsp olive oil

One Tbsp ground chipotle chili pepper

One Tbsp paprika

One Tbsp cumin

One Tbsp brown sugar

Salt and pepper to taste

Directions:

• Preheat your oven to 425°F and line your baking pan with parchment paper.

• In a small bowl, mix together chipotle, paprika, brown sugar, and cumin.

• Heat two Tbsp olive oil in a skillet over high heat. Season the meat with salt and cook for ten minutes, turning occasionally, until golden brown.

•   Transfer the roast to the baking pan and season with the prepared paprika-chipotle mixture.

•   In a large bowl, toss Brussels sprouts, onion, and potato with one Tbsp oil, salt and pepper. Then spread the veggies onto the same baking pan around the meat.

•   Place the pan in the oven and bake for twenty five minutes. Then remove the baking pan from the oven and transfer veggies to a bowl. Return the meat to the oven and bake for fifteen minutes.

•   Transfer the roast to a large platter and allow rest for ten minutes. Then slice the meat and divide into meal prep containers. Now add vegetables and let them cool down before storing in your fridge.

Time: 60 mins

Number of servings: 4

Ingredients:

One pound ground beef

One cup shredded mozzarella cheese

One cup ricotta cheese

One cup marinara sauce

Two zucchini, peeled and spiralized

Two Tbsp olive oil

Salt and pepper to taste

Directions:

- Preheat your oven to 350°F.

- Hcat the olive oil in your large skillet over medium heat. Add beef and cook for ten minutes, stirring constantly with a spatula. Then add marinara sauce and cook for three minutes more. Season with salt and pepper and let sit for fifteen minutes.

- In a small casserole dish, put layers in order: beef, zucchini noodles, ricotta cheese, beef, zoodles, ricotta, mozzarella cheese. Place this casserole dish in the oven and bake for thirty minutes. Then uncover lasagna and broil for three minutes to brown the top.

- Now slice the cooked lasagna and divide into meal prep containers. Let cool down before storing in your fridge.

Time: 20 mins (and three hours for marinating)

Number of servings: 4

Ingredients:

One pound top sirloin steak, cut into 1-inch pieces

Half cup soy sauce

One third cup olive oil

Quarter cup Worcestershire sauce

Two minced garlic cloves

Two Tbsp basil

One Tbsp parsley

Salt and pepper to taste

Directions:

• In a bowl, mix together soy sauce, olive oil, Worcestershire sauces, garlic, basil, parsley, salt, and pepper. Stir well to combine.

• Place the meat in a zip-lock plastic bag and add prepared marinade. Toss to coat and place the bag in your fridge for at least three hours.

• Heat a large skillet over medium-high heat. Remove beef pieces from marinade with a slotted spoon and cook for three minutes per side.

• Divide cooked steak pieces into meal prep containers and add veggies and side dish of your choice.

Quick and Easy Meatballs

Time: 20 mins

Number of servings: 4

Ingredients:

One pound ground beef

Two Tbsp parsley

One tsp onion powder

One tsp garlic powder

Salt and pepper to taste

Directions:

• Preheat your oven to 400°F and line your baking sheet with a parchment paper.

• In a large bowl, mix together all ingredients and stir well to combine. Divide the prepared mixture into eight parts and form each into a meatball.

• Place meatballs on the prepped baking sheet and bake for fifteen minutes.

• Transfer the cooked meatballs to your meal containers, evenly dividing. Let cool down before storing in your fridge. You can add spaghetti, mashed potatoes, or steamed rice as a side dish.

Time: 20 mins

Number of servings: 4

Ingredients:

One pound ground beef

Two cups diced Kabocha squash

Two sliced zucchini

Four tomatoes, quartered

Two Tbsp olive oil

Salt and pepper to taste

Directions:

• Preheat your oven to 425°F and line your baking sheet with a foil.

• Season the ground beef with salt and pepper and divide it into eight parts. Roll each part into ball and then flatten the ball into 0.5-inch thick patty.

• In a bowl, toss your veggies with the olive oil.

• Place burgers and veggies on the lined baking sheet. Bake for twenty minutes flipping burgers once halfway through cooking.

• Divide cooked burgers and veggies between your meal prep containers and let cool down before storing in your fridge.

Time: 30 mins

Number of servings: 6

Ingredients:

One pound lean ground beef

One 10-oz can of tomato soup

One cup salsa

One cup sliced mushrooms

One cup sliced onions

One cup sliced carrots

One cup frozen kernel corn

Half cup cheddar cheese

Half cup water

One minced garlic clove

Two Tbsp onion flakes

Two Tbsp olive oil

Half cup water

Directions:

•   Heat the olive oil in your large skillet over medium heat. Add beef and cook for ten minutes, stirring constantly with a spatula.

•   Add salsa, tomato soup, corn, water, and cook for five minutes more.

•   Now add mushrooms, carrots, onions, and cook for another five minutes.

•   Sprinkle with cheddar, garlic, and onion flakes. Stir well to combine and divide between your meal prep containers. Let cool down before storing in your fridge.

Time: 30 mins

Number of servings: 6

Ingredients:

Six 6-oz petite sirloin steaks

One and a half cup bleu cheese crumbles

Two Tbsp olive oil

Two tsp onion flakes

Two tsp kosher salt

Two tsp black pepper

One tsp garlic powder

One tsp thyme

One tsp rosemary

One tsp coriander

Directions:

•   In a small bowl, mix together onion flakes, kosher salt, black pepper, garlic powder, thyme, rosemary, and coriander. Season each steak with the prepared blend on both sides.

•   Heat the olive oil in your large skillet over high heat. Add meat and cook for four minutes on the first side.

•   Then flip steaks and top each with bleu cheese crumbles. Cook for another four minutes.

- Divide cooked steaks in your meal prep containers and let cool down before storing in your fridge.

Time: 60 mins

Number of servings: 4

Ingredients:

One pound sirloin steak, cut into bite-sized pieces

Four chopped red potatoes

Two sliced onion

Four Tbsp olive oil

Three tsp garlic powder

Salt and pepper to taste

Directions:

- Preheat your oven to 350°F.

- In a large bowl, mix together meat, potatoes, and onion. Add olive oil and toss to coat.

- Transfer the meat-potatoes mixture to a baking dish and bake for forty five minutes.

- Divide cooked beef with onion and potatoes between your meal prep containers and let cool down before storing in your fridge.

Time: 40 mins

Number of servings: 4

Ingredients:

One pound lean ground beef

One cup brown rice

Four boiled eggs, peeled and halved

Four cups chopped spinach

Two sliced green onions

Two minced garlic cloves

Three Tbsp olive oil

Quarter cup brown sugar

Quarter cup soy sauce

One Tbsp grated ginger

Two tsp sesame oil

Half tsp sriracha sauce

A pinch of sesame seeds

Directions:

• Cook brown rice according to the info on the package and set aside.

• In a small bowl, whisk together soy sauce, sesame oil, ginger, and sriracha sauce.

•	Heat the olive oil in your skillet over medium-high heat. Add garlic and cook for one minute, stirring frequently. Then add ground beef and cook for seven minutes, stirring constantly with a spatula.

•	Add soy sauce, spinach, and soy sauce mixture, and cook for three minutes.

•	Divide cooked brown rice between your meal prep containers. Add eggs, ground beef mixture, and top with green onions and sesame seeds. Let cool down before storing in your fridge.

Time: 60 mins

Number of servings: 4

Ingredients:

One and a half pound lean ground beef

Eight halved and seeded bell peppers

One diced onion

Five minced garlic cloves

One 12-oz can of tomato paste

One 6-oz can of hot diced green chiles

Three Tbsp chopped cilantro

One Tbsp olive oil

One Tbsp garlic powder

Half tsp paprika

Half tsp ground red pepper

Salt and pepper to taste

Directions:

- Preheat your oven to 350°F.

- Heat olive oil in a skillet over medium high heat. Add onion and sauté for five minutes. Then add garlic and cook for just one minute.

- Now add ground beef and cook for ten minutes, stirring constantly with a spatula.

- Add tomato paste, green chiles, garlic powder, paprika, red pepper, salt, and pepper. Stir and cook for additional two minutes.

- Spoon ground beef mixture into the pepper halves and place them in a baking dish. Cover with a foil and transfer in the oven.

- Bake for twenty minutes, then uncover and cook for ten minutes more.

- Divide stuffed bell peppers between meal prep containers and sprinkle with cilantro. Let cool down before storing in your fridge.

Pork has high protein containing, which is helpful to form and maintain your muscle and strengthen the immune. On the other hand, pork has high calories and fat content too. Thus, it's not recommended to consume the pork over when you are not exercising and less moving.

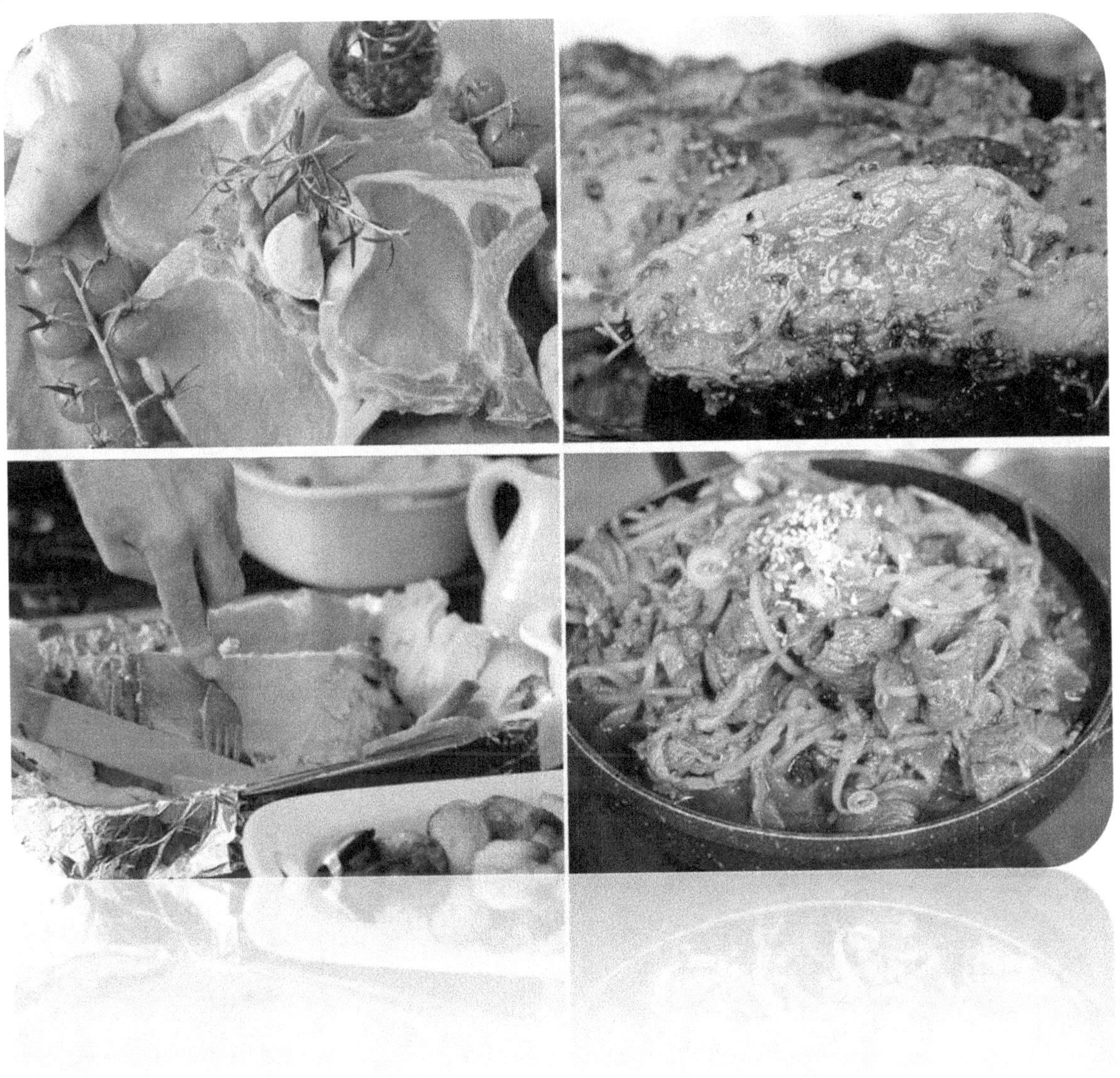

Pork is a nutrient-dense food; it's rich in Zinc, Phosphorous, Potassium, Niacin, vitamin B6, Riboflavin, and Thiamin. Thiamin is a key vitamin for protein, carb, and fat metabolism. Animal proteins are good for providing us with Thiamin, and pork is the best source among the choices.

High level of collagen is another nutritional benefit of consuming pork. Eating collagen may help to hydrate your skin, prevent joint deterioration, and minimize some signs of aging.

Time: 45 mins

Number of servings: 6

Ingredients:

Six pork chops, bone-in

Two pounds baby potatoes

Three Tbsp olive oil

One 1-oz package of ranch salad dressing and seasoning mix

One Tbsp chopped fresh parsley

One Tbsp dry oregano

One tsp ground black pepper

One tsp smoked paprika

Salt to taste

Directions:

• Preheat your oven to 400°F and line your baking sheet with a foil.

• In a small bowl, mix together the ranch seasoning, oregano, ground black pepper, paprika, and salt.

• Place pork chops and potatoes on the baking sheet, cover with the olive oil and toss well. Then sprinkle with the prepared seasoning mix.

• Place the baking sheet in the oven and bake for forty minutes.

- Divide cooked pork chops and potatoes between your meal prep containers. Garnish with chopped parsley and let cool down before storing in your fridge.

Herb-Crusted Pork Chops

Time: 30 mins

Number of servings: 4

Ingredients:

Four pork chops, boneless and fat trimmed

Half cup whole wheat Panko breadcrumbs

Two Tbsp Dijon mustard

One Tbsp olive oil

One Tbsp chopped parsley

One Tbsp chopped thyme

Salt and pepper to taste

Directions:

- Preheat your oven to 450°F.

- In your large bowl, mix together the breadcrumbs, parsley, thyme, salt, and pepper.

- Cover each pork chop with the mustard evenly and then dredge in the prepared dry mix.

- Heat the olive oil in your skillet over medium-high heat. Add pork and cook for two minutes per side, until golden brown.

- Now flip pork chops over and place the skillet in the oven for ten minutes.

- Divide cooked pork chops in meal prep containers. Add a side dish and veggies of choice and let cool down before storing in your fridge.

Time: 30 mins

Number of servings: 4

Ingredients:

Four center cut pork chops

Two bell peppers, cut into strips

Three sliced garlic cloves

One Tbsp olive oil

Two tsp balsamic vinegar

Two tsp chopped fresh rosemary

Salt and pepper to taste

Directions:

•   Heat the olive oil in your skillet over medium-high heat. Season pork chops with salt and pepper, and add to the skillet. Cook for seven minutes.

•   Now reduce heat to medium and flip pork chops over. Add bell peppers, garlic, one tsp rosemary, and cook for ten minutes.

•   Drizzle the meat and peppers with balsamic vinegar and top with reserved rosemary.

•   Divide cooked pork chops in meal prep containers. Add a side dish and veggies of choice and let cool down before storing in your fridge.

Time: 50 mins (and three hours for marinating)

Number of servings: 4

Ingredients:

Two pounds pork chops, boneless

Three sweet potatoes, cubed

Two onions, sliced

Juice of two oranges

Six Tbsp molasses

Five Tbsp olive oil

Three Tbsp dried basil

Three tsp garlic powder

Three tsp cinnamon

One tsp allspice

One tsp honey

Salt and pepper to taste

Directions:

•   Place pork chops in a zip-lock plastic bag. Add molasses, juice of one orange, basil, salt, and pepper. Seal and shake to coat pork chops evenly. Marinate in your fridge for at least three hours.

- In a large bowl, mix together remaining orange juice, four Tbsp olive oil, garlic, cinnamon, allspice, honey, salt, and pepper. Then add sweet potatoes and toss to coat.

- Heat reserved one Tbsp olive oil in a skillet over medium heat. Add onions, sweet potatoes, and cook for ten minutes, stirring often.

- Add pork chops in the middle of the skillet and cook for two minutes per side. Then add marinating juices and carefully transfer the skillet in the oven, and bake for twenty minutes.

- Divide cooked pork chops with sweet potatoes in your meal prep containers, and let cool down before storing in your fridge.

Pork Cutlets with Beans and Bell Peppers

Time: 50 mins

Number of servings: 8

Ingredients:

Three pounds pork cutlets, pounded ¼-inch thick

Two 15-oz cans of cannellini beans, rinsed

Four sliced bell peppers

Four sliced shallots

One cup kalamata olives, pitted and halved

One cup chopped parsley

Four Tbsp olive oil

Four Tbsp red wine vinegar

Salt and pepper to taste

Directions:

•   Season each pork cutlet with salt and pepper on both sides. Heat one Tbsp olive oil in a skillet over medium high heat. Add pork and cook for three minutes per side and then transfer to a platter. Cook all meat in three butches, adding oil every time.

•   Now heat the reserved one Tbsp olive oil in another skillet over medium high heat. Add shallots, bell peppers, salt, and pepper. Cook for five minutes, stirring occasionally.

•   Add the beans, parsley, olives, and vinegar to veggies and stir well to combine. Cook for additional two minutes.

- Divide cooked pork cutlets in your meal prep containers, and top with the vegetable mixture. Let cool down before storing in your fridge.

Dijon Pork with Fruits and Quinoa

Time: 20 mins

Number of servings: 8

Ingredients:

Three pounds pork tenderloin, cut into medallions

Four cups cooked quinoa

Two chopped onions

Two diced apples

One cup diced mango

Half cup water

Four Tbsp Dijon mustard

Two Tbsp honey

Two Tbsp olive oil

Directions:

- In a bowl, mix together water, honey, and Dijon mustard.

- Heat olive oil in a skillet over medium heat. Add onion and sauté for two minutes.

- Add pork and cook for three minutes per side. Then add apples, mango, and Dijon mustard mixture, and cook for three minutes, until apple is tender.

- Divide cooked quinoa between your meal prep containers, and top with meat and fruits. Let cool down before storing in your fridge.

Time: 30 mins

Number of servings: 4

Ingredients:

Two pounds lean ground pork

One 8-oz can of water chestnuts, drained and chopped

Five shredded carrots

Two diced onions

Two cups bean sprouts

One cup chopped cilantro

Half cup chopped green onions

Two minced garlic cloves

Half cup soy sauce

Quarter cup rice vinegar

Quarter cup honcy

Two Tbsp Dijon mustard

Two Tbsp peanut butter

Two Tbsp sesame oil

Two Tbsp rice vinegar

Two Tbsp water

Two tsp grated ginger

Two tsp sriracha sauce

Salt and pepper to taste

Large Bibb lettuce leaves

Directions:

•	Heat a large skillet over medium high heat. Add ground pork, onion, salt, pepper and cook for ten minutes, stirring often with a spatula.

•	Add ginger, garlic and cook for just one minute. Then add quarter cup soy sauce, sesame oil, rice vinegar, peanut butter, water, and one tsp sriracha. Stir well to combine and add water chestnuts and green onion. Cook for two additional minutes.

•	In a small bowl, mix together reserved quarter cup soy sauce, one tsp sriracha sauce, honey, and Dijon mustard.

•	Spoon pork mixture into lettuce leaf. Then top with carrots, bean sprouts, and cilantro. Drizzle with prepared sauce and wrap.

•	Divide pork lettuce wraps in your meal prep containers, and let cool down before storing in your fridge.

Time: 50 mins

Number of servings: 4

Ingredients:

One pound pork tenderloin

Half pound baby potatoes, quartered

One cup baby carrots

One Tbsp olive oil

One tsp dried thyme

Half tsp paprika

Salt and pepper to taste

Directions:

•   Preheat your oven to 375°F and line your baking sheet with a foil.

•   Season the tenderloin with salt and pepper on both sides. Then place meat at the center of the baking sheet.

•   In a large bowl, mix together olive oil, thyme, paprika, salt, and pepper. Add carrots and potatoes, and toss to coat.

•   Then transfer carrots and potatoes to the baking sheet and bake for thirty-five minutes. Remove the pork with veggies from the oven and let sit for five minutes.

•   Slice cooked pork tenderloin and divide between meal prep containers. Add potatoes, carrots, and let cool down before storing in your fridge.

Time: 9 hours 40 mins

Number of servings: 12

Ingredients:

Five pounds pork shoulder

Three Tbsp paprika

Three Tbsp coarse sea salt

One Tbsp dry mustard

One Tbsp brown sugar

One Tbsp garlic powder

Directions:

•   In a small bowl, mix together paprika, coarse sea salt, dry mustard, brown sugar, garlic powder. Season the pork with prepared spice bend. Then cover and place in your fridge for at least one hour.

•   Preheat your oven to 300°F.

•   Put marinated pork in a roasting pan and roast for six hours, until it's falling apart.

•   When the meat is ready, take it out of the oven and transfer to a large platter. Allow the cooked pork to rest for ten minutes.

•   While the prepared meat is still warm, pull it with two forks. Put the shredded pork in a large container and let cool down before storing in your fridge. You can use it for prepping a wide variety of healthy meals.

Time: 50 mins

Number of servings: 4

Ingredients:

Four cups shredded pork

Two heads of broccoli, chopped

Two diced sweet potatoes

One cup BBQ sauce

Three Tbsp olive oil

Two tsp paprika

Two tsp garlic powder

One tsp onion powder

Salt and pepper to taste

Directions:

•   Preheat your oven to 400°F and line your baking sheet with a foil.

•   In a large bowl, mix together olive oil, paprika, garlic powder, onion powder, salt, and pepper. Add potatoes, broccoli, and toss to coat.

•   Then place veggies on the baking sheet and bake for forty minutes.

- Divide cooked vegetables between meal prep containers. Add shredded pork and drizzle with BBQ sauce. Let cool down before storing in your fridge.

Creamy Pulled Pork Pasta

Time: 40 mins

Number of servings: 6

Ingredients:

Four cups shredded pork

One 12-oz package spaghetti pasta

One 12-oz can of diced tomatoes

One and a half cup cheddar cheese, shredded

Half cup cream cheese

Half cup BBQ sauce

Half cup chopped green onions

One Tbsp olive oil

Directions:

• Cook the pasta according to the info on the package and set aside.

• Preheat your oven to 400°F.

• Warm the olive oil in the ovenproof skillet over low heat. Add pork, tomatoes, BBQ sauce, and cream cheese. Stir and cook for one minute, until cream cheese is melty.

• Then add cooked spaghetti, green onions, and stir until combined. Spread the pasta evenly in the skillet and top with shredded cheddar.

- Transfer the skillet to the oven and bake for fifteen minutes. When ready, slice the pasta and divide between your meal prep containers. Let cool down before storing in your fridge.

Most veggies are naturally low in calories, so you can consume your hearty meal without worrying about counting calories. Veggies, lentils, and grains nourish beneficial bacteria in the gut, due to the fiber content. Also, soluble fiber helps you to reduce blood cholesterol. And lowering cholesterol levels reduces the risk of stroke and heart disease by keeping blood vessels clean.

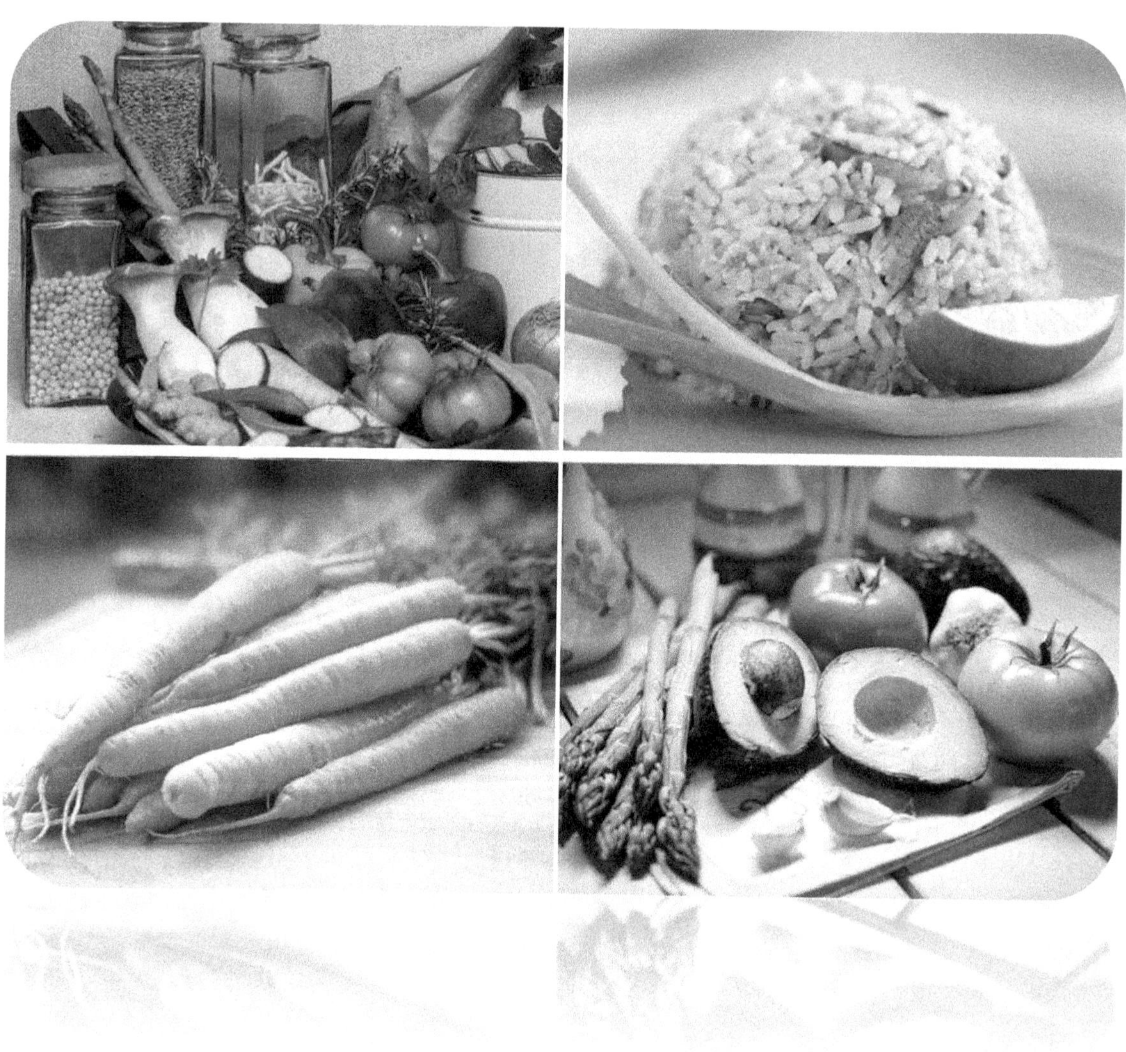

A plant-based diet is rich in vitamins C and A, potassium, folic acid and more. Although lentils, vegetables, and whole grains include all these beneficial nutrients, they are still low in fat and calories. For example, one cup of cooked lentils contains about 250 calories only and leaves you satisfied and feeling full. On the flip side, plant-based foods provide steady energy flow due to complex carbohydrates.

Time: 30 mins

Number of servings: 4

Ingredients:

Two cups cooked chickpeas

One cup quinoa

One 7-oz pack of feta

Two cups diced tomatoes

One chopped onion

Two diced cucumbers

One cup water

Half cup olive oil

Two Tbsp lemon juice

Two Tbsp honey

Two Tbsp tahini

Salt and pepper to taste

Directions:

• Cook quinoa according to the info on the package.

• Meanwhile, divide chickpeas, feta, and veggies between meal prep containers.

• In a bowl, mix together honey, lemon juice, tahini, and olive oil. Stir well to combine.

- Divide cooked quinoa in prep containers and let cool down before storing in your fridge. Store the prepared dressing in 3-oz mini containers, and add to it to bowl just before eating.

Time: 60 mins

Number of servings: 8

Ingredients:

Four cups cooked and cooled rice

Six eggs

Two cups diced green beans

Two diced onions

Two peeled and chopped carrots

One chopped bell pepper

Quarter cup soy sauce

Three Tbsp grated ginger

Two Tbsp olive oil

One Tbsp sesame oil

One Tbsp sesame seeds

Salt and pepper to taste

Directions:

•   Heat one Tbsp olive oil in a large skillet over medium heat. Beat the eggs and cook, scrambling, for five minutes, until cooked through. Then transfer to a platter.

•   Add the reserved Tbsp of olive oil, onions, ginger, and sauté for three minutes. Then add green beans, bell pepper, carrots and cook for additional five minutes.

- Now add the sesame oil, soy sauce, and cooked rice. Stir well to combine.

- Finally, add eggs and season with salt and pepper. Then divide in meal prep containers and top with sesame seeds. Let cool down before storing in your fridge.

Time: 30 mins

Number of servings: 4

Ingredients:

One pound firm tofu

Two cups sliced baby bella mushrooms

Two cups chopped kale

One chopped onion

One chopped bell pepper

One minced garlic clove

One Tbsp olive oil

Two tsp curry powder

One tsp turmeric

One tsp cumin

Salt and pepper to taste

Directions:

•   Heat the olive oil in your skillet over medium heat. Add garlic and cook for a minute. Then add mushrooms, onion, bell pepper and cook, stirring occasionally, for five minutes.

•   Now add tofu and break it up with a spatula. Add cumin, curry, turmeric, salt, pepper and stir well to combine. Cook, stirring occasionally, for seven minutes.

- Divide the cooked scramble into meal prep containers and top with chopped kale. Let cool down before storing in your fridge.

Time: 40 mins

Number of servings: 4

Ingredients:

One 15-oz can of black beans

One 15-oz can of pumpkin

One 15-oz can of diced tomatoes

One 15-oz can of corn

Two cups of chopped kale

One chopped onion

One chopped bell pepper

One minced garlic clove

Two cups water

Two Tbsp olive oil

One Tbsp cumin

Two tsp cinnamon

One tsp chili powder

A pinch of cayenne pepper

Salt and pepper to taste

Directions:

- Heat the olive oil in your large pot over medium heat. Add onion, garlic, and sauté for a minute. Then add pumpkin, tomatoes with juices, and water. Stir well to combine.

- Now add black beans, corn, bell pepper, cumin, cinnamon, chili powder, and cayenne pepper. Stir again and bring the mixture to a boil.

- Reduce heat to low and simmer for fifteen minutes. Stir in prepped kale and season with salt and pepper. Cook for another fifteen minutes.

- Divide cooked chili into meal prep containers and let cool down before storing in your fridge.

Time: 60 mins

Number of servings: 4

Ingredients:

One 10-oz package of whole grain pasta

Half peeled and cubed butternut squash

One 8-oz pack of baby bella mushrooms, sliced

Two minced garlic cloves

Two cups chopped kale

Two cups veggie stock

One cup milk

Two Tbsp coconut oil

Salt and pepper to taste

Directions:

•   Cook the whole grain pasta according to the info on the package and set aside.

•   Heat one Tbsp coconut oil in a large skillet over medium heat. Add butternut squash, one clove of garlic, and veggie stock. Stir well and bring to a boil. Reduce the heat to low and simmer for twenty minutes.

•   Transfer cooked squash to your blender. Add milk and blend until smooth. Season with salt and pepper.

•	In the same skillet, heat the remaining one Tbsp coconut oil over medium heat. Add mushrooms, garlic, and cook for five minutes. Then add kale and cook for another five minutes.

•	Remove from the heat and add squash and pasta to the skillet. Stir well to combine and divide between meal prep containers. Let cool down before storing in your fridge.

Time: 80 mins

Number of servings: 4

Ingredients:

One cup white rice

One cup rinsed and drained lentils

One cup rinsed and drained chickpeas

One 15-oz can of diced tomatoes

One 15-oz can of coconut milk

One chopped onion

One sliced lime

Two minced garlic cloves

One Tbsp coconut oil

One Tbsp garam masala

Two tsp curry powder

Two tsp cumin

One tsp minced ginger

Salt and pepper to taste

Directions:

•   Cook the rice according to the info on the package and set aside.

- Heat the coconut oil in a large skillet over high heat. Add tomatoes, onion, and garlic and stir. Then reduce heat to low medium and cook for ten minutes.

- Now add lentils, chickpeas, ginger, and spices. Stir well to combine.

- Pour in coconut milk and water. Stir and bring the mixture to a boil. Then reduce heat, cover, and simmer for thirty minutes.

- Divide cooked rice into meal prep containers, add curry, and top with lime slices. Let cool down before storing in your fridge.

Burrito Bowl with Black Beans

Time: 20 mins

Number of servings: 4

Ingredients:

Two cups cooked brown rice

One 15-oz can of black beans, drained and rinsed

One cup canned corn

One cup shredded cheddar cheese

One cup chopped kale

One chopped tomato

Juice of one lime

Two Tbsp olive oil

One tsp cumin

Salt and pepper to taste

Directions:

•   Heat the olive oil in your skillet over medium heat. Add black beans, corn, cumin, salt, and pepper. Cook for five minutes, stirring occasionally.

•   Add chopped tomatoes, stir, and cook for three minutes more. Then remove from the heat, add cheese, and set aside.

•   Divide cooked rice between your meal prep containers, add kale, and top with tomato mixture. Drizzle with the juice of lime and let cool down before storing in your fridge.

Time: 30 mins

Number of servings: 6

Ingredients:

Two cups French lentils

Two chopped cucumbers

One cup kalamata olives, pitted and halved

One cup crumbled feta cheese

Half cup chopped fresh mint

Two minced garlic cloves

Six Tbsp olive oil

Two Tbsp sherry vinegar

Two bay leaves

Two tsp whole-grain mustard

Salt to taste

Directions:

• In a large pot, mix together French lentils, garlic, and bay leaves. Cover with water and bring to a boil over high heat. Then reduce the heat and simmer for fifteen minutes, until tender. Drain the water, discard bay leaves and garlic, and let cool down.

• In your small bowl, whisk together sherry vinegar, mustard, and olive oil. Stir well to combine.

- In a large bowl, mix together cooked French lentils, olives, cucumbers, and mint. Pour prepared vinaigrette over salad and toss to coat.

- Divide salad between meal prep containers, and top with crumbled feta cheese. You can store this salad in your fridge for up to four days.

Lentil Shepherd's Pie with Mushrooms and Sweet Potatoes

Time: 100 mins

Number of servings: 6

Ingredients:

One cup green lentils, rinsed

One pound baby bella mushrooms, chopped

Four sweet potatoes

One cup steel-cut oats

One chopped onion

One chopped carrot

One chopped celery stalk

One minced garlic clove

Five cups water

One cup vegetable stock

Quarter cup dry red wine

One Tbsp soy sauce

One Tbsp olive oil

One Tbsp tomato paste

One tsp smoked paprika

One bay leaf

Salt and pepper to taste

Directions:

- Preheat your oven to 400°F. Place sweet potatoes on a baking sheet and bake for one hour.

- Meanwhile, in a medium saucepan, mix together lentils, oats, bay leaf, and salt. Add five cups of water and bring to a boil over high heat. Then reduce heat and simmer for twenty minutes, stirring occasionally. When ready, drain the mixture and discard the bay leaf.

- Warm the olive oil in a large pot over medium-high heat. Add mushrooms, carrot, onion, celery, garlic, and cook for ten minutes, stirring occasionally.

- Reduce heat to medium and add lentil-oat mixture, vegetable stock, wine, tomato paste, soy sauce, and paprika. Cook for five minutes. Then remove the pot from heat and season with salt and pepper.

- When sweet potatoes are ready, reduce oven temperature to 350°F. Peel sweet potatoes and mash them into a smooth paste.

- Evenly spread the lentil-mushroom mixture into a baking dish. Then top with the sweet potato mixture and smooth with a spatula. Bake for thirty minutes.

- Slice and divide cooked shepherd's pie between your meal prep containers. Let cool down before storing in your fridge.

Time: 50 mins

Number of servings: 6

Ingredients:

Two pounds Brussels sprouts, trimmed and halved

Two cups quinoa, rinsed

One cup green lentils, rinsed

One chopped onion

One minced garlic clove

Two cups vegetable stock

Four Tbsp olive oil

Two Tbsp honey

Two tsp cumin

Two tsp coriander

Half tsp turmeric

Half tsp cinnamon

Salt and pepper to taste

Directions:

• Preheat your oven to 400°F. Place the sprouts on a baking sheet, drizzle with two Tbsp olive oil, and season with salt and pepper. Transfer the baking sheet in the oven and roast for thirty minutes.

•   Meanwhile, bring a large saucepan of water to a boil over high heat. Then add the lentils, reduce heat to low, and simmer for twenty five minutes. Drain and season with salt and pepper.

•   When Brussels sprouts are ready, remove from the oven and drizzle with the honey.

•   Heat the remaining two Tbsp olive oil in a large saucepan over medium heat. Add the onions, garlic, and sauté for two minutes. Then add quinoa, coriander, cinnamon, cumin, and turmeric. Stir to coat grains with the spices.

•   Now add vegetable stock, cover, and cook for twenty minutes. Then remove from the heat and let sit for five minutes. Add cooked lentils and gently fluff the mixture with a fork.

•   Divide cooked lentil-quinoa pilaf between meal prep containers. Top with the honey-roasted Brussels sprouts, and let cool down before storing in your fridge.

Time: 20 mins

Number of servings: 4

Ingredients:

Two cups boiled white beans

Four hard-boiled eggs, halved

Two chopped bell peppers

Two sliced red onions

One chopped tomato

One chopped cucumber

Two cups water

Quarter cup chopped green onions

Quarter cup chopped fresh dill

Quarter cup chopped parsley

Two Tbsp olive oil

One Tbsp lemon juice

One tsp vinegar

Salt to taste

Directions:

•   In your large bowl, mix together the beans, tomatoes, cucumbers, green peppers, green onions, dill, parsley, and olive oil.

- In your small saucepan, pour water and bring to a boil over medium-high heat. Add red onions and blanch for a minute. Then transfer them to the bowl with cold water for two minutes. Then drain and set aside.

- In a small bowl, mix together lemon juice, vinegar, and salt. Pour prepared mixture over drained red onions and let sit for five minutes.

- Transfer red onions to the bowl with salad and stir well to combine. Divide white beans salad between your meal prep containers. Top with halved eggs, and let cool down before storing in your fridge.

Time: 80 mins

Number of servings: 4

Ingredients:

Two 8-oz packages of chickpea pasta spirals

One cup brown lentils

Two shredded carrots

One sliced onion

One sliced bell pepper

Four minced garlic cloves

One 6-oz can of tomato paste

One cup halved cherry tomatoes

Half cup grated parmesan cheese

Four cups water

Four Tbsp olive oil

One Tbsp miso paste

One tsp sugar

Salt and pepper to taste

Directions:

•   Cook the chickpea pasta according to the info on the package and set aside.

•   Warm the olive oil in a large skillet over medium high heat. Add onions and sauté for five minutes. Then add the carrots, bell pepper, salt, sugar, and cook, stirring occasionally, for fifteen minutes, until caramelized.

•   Now add the tomato paste, garlic, and cook for additional three minutes.

•   Add the water, lentils, miso, and bring to a boil. Reduce the heat and cook for thirty minutes, stirring occasionally. Then add cherry tomatoes and stir well.

•   Divide cooked pasta between your meal prep containers. Top with lentil Bolognese and grated parmesan. Let cool down before storing in your fridge.

Time: 30 mins

Number of servings: 4

Ingredients:

Two cups quinoa, rinsed

Two sliced bell peppers

Three sliced scallions

Two peeled and grated carrots

Two chopped cucumber

Three cups water

Half cup chopped cilantro

Half cup lime juice

Quarter cup chopped basil

Three Tbsp sugar

Three Tbsp olive oil

Two Tbsp fish sauce

One tsp salt

Half tsp crushed red pepper flakes

Directions:

• Place quinoa in a medium saucepan. Add water, salt, and bring to a boil over medium high heat. Then reduce heat to low, cover, and cook for fifteen minutes, until water is absorbed. Then transfer to a bowl and let cool down.

• In a medium bowl, mix together lime juice, fish sauce, olive oil, sugar, and red pepper. Stir well, until sugar is dissolved.

• In a large bowl, mix together quinoa, bell peppers, cucumbers, carrots, scallions, cilantro, and basil. Then add prepared vinaigrette and stir well to combine.

• Divide the salad between your meal prep containers, and let cool down before storing in your fridge.

Time: 30 mins

Number of servings: 4

Ingredients:

One 18-oz tube of polenta, opened and cut into chunks

Four cups kale

One sliced red onion

Two cups vegetable stock

Six Tbsp olive oil

Half Tbsp garlic powder

Salt and pepper to taste

Directions:

•   Place the polenta into a medium pot and turn to medium-high heat. Cook, adding a half cup of vegetable stock at a time and stirring continuously, until polenta is creamy. Then remove your pot from the heat and set aside.

•   Heat three Tbsp olive oil in a skillet over medium heat. Add red onions and cook for eight minutes, stirring occasionally. Then season with salt and pepper, and set aside.

•   Heat reserved three Tbsp olive oil in the same skillet. Add kale and sauté for two minutes. Then season with salt, garlic powder, and set aside.

•   Divide cooked polenta between your meal prep containers. Top with kale and caramelized onions. Let cool down before storing in your fridge.

Vegetable Enchilada

Time: 50 mins

Number of servings: 4

Ingredients:

One 15-oz can of black beans, drained and rinsed

One 19-oz can of enchilada sauce

One cup corn kernels

One cup shredded cheese

Six chopped up corn tortillas

One diced summer squash

One diced zucchini

One diced bell pepper

Half onion, diced

One Tbsp olive oil

One tsp paprika

One tsp cumin

One tsp garlic powder

Salt and pepper to taste

Directions:

- Preheat your oven to 375°F.

- Warm olive oil in a skillet over medium heat. Add onion, bell pepper, summer squash, zucchini, corn kernels, and cook for seven minutes.

- Then add black beans, paprika, cumin, garlic powder, salt, and pepper. Stir well and cook for additional two minutes.

- In a medium baking dish, add half cup enchilada sauce to the bottom. Then top with two cups vegetable mixture, one cup chopped corn tortillas, half cup cheese and then another half cup enchilada sauce. Repeat all process one more time ending with a layer of shredded cheese on top.

- Place the baking dish in the oven and bake for twenty minutes, until cheese is melted.

- Remove from the oven, slice the cooked enchilada, and divide into your meal prep containers. Let cool down before storing in your fridge.

Time: 40 mins (and one hour for marinating)

Number of servings: 4

Ingredients:

One 19-oz package of extra firm tofu, drained and cut into eight parts

Three minced garlic cloves

Juice of one lemon

Juice of half orange

Half cup water

Two Tbsp soy sauce

One Tbsp grated ginger

One Tbsp sesame oil

One Tbsp rice wine vinegar

Black pepper to taste

Directions:

•   In your large bowl, mix together lemon juice, orange juice, water, soy sauce, vinegar, sesame oil, ginger, garlic, and black pepper. Stir well to combine and add tofu slices. Toss to coat, cover, and marinate in your fridge at least for one hour.

• Preheat your oven to 190°F.

- Place the marinated tofu in a baking dish and pour over remaining marinade. Cover the baking dish with a foil and bake for twenty minutes. Then flip up tofu and cook for additional fifteen minutes uncovered.

- Divide cooked tofu between your meal prep containers, and let cool down before storing in your fridge.

Simple Vegetable Fried Rice

Time: 30 mins

Number of servings: 4

Ingredients:

One cup brown rice

Two cups edamame

One cup green peas

One cup corn

Two diced carrots

Two diced stalks celery

Two chopped bell peppers

One chopped onion

Half cup soy sauce

Half cup chopped green onions

Two Tbsp olive oil

One tsp grated ginger

Salt and pepper to taste

Directions:

• Cook the brown rice according to the info on the package.

• Warm the olive oil in a skillet over medium heat. Add onion, bell pepper, celery, carrot, and cook for five minutes, stirring occasionally.

- Now add rice, edamame, green peas, ginger, corn, and soy sauce. Stir well to combine and cook for another five minutes. Season with salt and pepper and remove from the heat.

- Divide cooked rice with veggies in meal prep containers, and let cool down before storing in your fridge.

Time: 20 mins

Number of servings: 4

Ingredients:

One 8-oz package of ramen noodle, cooked

Five sliced scallion stalks

Three cups shredded red cabbage

One cup grated carrot

Quarter cup chopped almonds

Quarter cup smooth peanut butter

Juice of half lime

Three Tbsp apple cider vinegar

Three Tbsp water

Two Tbsp soy sauce

Two Tbsp maple syrup

Half tsp onion powder

Half tsp garlic powder

Directions:

•   In a large bowl, mix together cooked ramen noodles, cabbage, carrots, scallions, and almonds. Stir well to combine.

- In your smaller bowl, whisk together peanut butter, lime juice, vinegar, maple syrup, soy sauce, garlic powder, onion powder, and water.

- Add prepared dressing to the salad and stir well to combine. Divide the salad between meal prep containers, and store them in your fridge.

Time: 30 mins

Number of servings: 4

Ingredients:

One chopped small head cauliflower, florets are halved

Four minced garlic cloves

Half cup soy sauce

Quarter cup honey

Quarter cup rice vinegar

Quarter cup water

One and a half Tbsp cornstarch

Two tsp sesame oil

Half tsp powdered ginger

Sesame seeds for garnish

Directions:

•   Preheat your oven to 400°F and line your baking sheet with a parchment paper.

•   Place cauliflower on the baking sheet in a single layer and bake for ten minutes.

•   Meanwhile, in a saucepan, whisk together soy sauce, honey, vinegar, garlic, sesame oil, and ginger. Warm the mixture over medium-high heat.

•   In your small bowl, whisk together cornstarch and water. Stir prepared thickener into the saucepan, when it boils. Reduce the heat to medium and cook for two minutes, stirring frequently.

•   Flip up cauliflower florets and cook for another ten minutes.

•   Divide baked cauliflower between meal prep containers, and pour prepared sauce over florets. Let cool down before storing in your fridge.

Time: 45 mins

Number of servings: 4

Ingredients:

One and a half cup farro

One 10-oz pack of lacinato kale, chopped

One 15-oz package of feta cheese, crumbled

One cup sliced artichoke hearts

One cup diced cucumber

One cup sliced bell peppers

Half red onion, sliced

Quarter cup olives, pitted and chopped

Two cups vegetable stock

Juice of two lemons

Quarter cup tahini

One bunch parsley, chopped

Directions:

•   Place farro in a large pot and pour over vegetable stock. Bring to a boil, then reduce the heat and simmer for thirty minutes. Then drain and set aside.

•   In a large bowl, mix together kale, and parsley. Stir well to combine thoroughly.

- Add farro, feta, artichoke, cucumber, bell peppers, olives, and onion. Stir well to combine.

- Divide the salad between meal prep containers, and store them in your fridge.

Time: 75 mins

Number of servings: 4

Ingredients:

One cup wild rice

One pound beets, peeled and halved

One cup toasted pecans, chopped

Two cups water

Three Tbsp olive oil

One Tbsp Dijon mustard

One Tbsp maple syrup

One Tbsp apple cider vinegar

Five sprigs fresh thyme

Salt and pepper to taste

Directions:

- Preheat your oven to 425°F

- Place beets in a large baking dish. Drizzle with one Tbsp olive oil and toss to coat. Cover the dish with foil and bake for one hour.

- Meanwhile, place the wild rice in a saucepan and add two cups water. Bring to a boil, then simmer for forty minutes.

- In a small bowl, whisk together reserved two Tbsp olive oil, apple cider vinegar, Dijon mustard, maple syrup, salt, and pepper. Stir well to combine.

- Cut cooked beets into bite-sized pieces and add them to the rice. Drizzle with the prepared maple-Dijon mixture and stir well to combine.

- Divide the rice with beets between meal prep containers, and top with the pecans. Let cool down before storing in your fridge.

Actually, snacking is not necessary, if you have three well-balanced meals a day. However, in case you have that snacking habit, you should plan your snacks ahead. Meal prep helps you avoid the making decisions in the moment of hunger pangs. So, you will eat something healthy, not just sugar and empty calories.

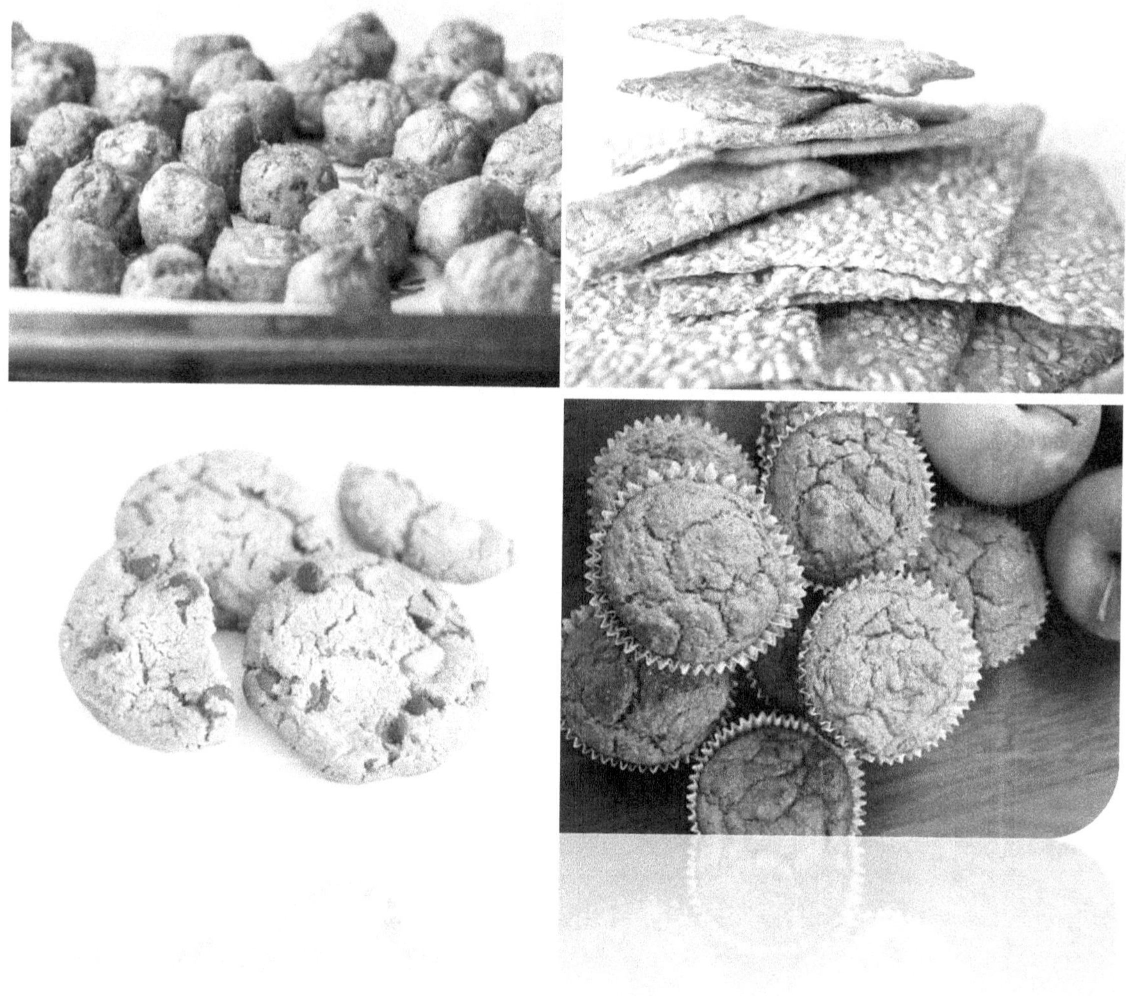

Of course, grabbing some fruit, veggie, nuts, and seeds is the easiest and quick option. It's like grabbing a candy bar, but the fruit is a nature's candy! The key to healthy snacking is planning ahead. And when you get bored with these simple options, try something new from recipes below.

Time: 30 mins

Number of servings: 8

Ingredients:

Four eggs

Half cup frozen blueberries

Half cup coconut flour

Half cup water

Quarter cup melted butter

Quarter cup Swerve Sweetener

One tsp baking powder

Half tsp salt

Half tsp vanilla extract

A pinch of cinnamon

Directions:

•   Preheat your oven to 325°F and grease a mini muffin 24-cup tin.

•   In your blender, mix together the eggs, sweetener, vanilla extract, and blend until smooth.

•   Now add melted butter, coconut flour, baking powder, salt, and cinnamon, and blend again. Let it sit for just five minutes, then add water and blend once again.

•	Divide the mixture among the muffin cups and add five blueberries to each. Transfer to the oven and bake for twenty-five minutes.

•	Divide cooked blueberries pancake bites between meal prep containers and let cool down before storing in your fridge.

Time: 80 mins

Number of servings: 12

Ingredients:

One cup of whole dates, pitted

One cup mix of dried apricots, prunes, and raisins

One cup mix of almonds, walnuts, and sunflower seeds

One Tbsp raw honey

Two tsp grated ginger

Half tsp cinnamon

Directions:

•   Place all your ingredients in your food processor and pulse for two minutes.

•   Line a large pancake pan with cellophane. Dispense the prepared mixture evenly and press until flat. Then cover and refrigerate for one hour.

•   Cut the mixture into twelve healthy energy bars. Divide in meal prep containers and store in your fridge.

Time: 35 mins

Number of servings: 12

Ingredients:

Half cup mashed bananas

Half cup unsweetened coconut flakes

Quarter cup dark chocolate chips

Two Tbsp coconut flour

Directions:

• Preheat your oven to 355°F and line a baking sheet with a parchment paper.

• In a bowl, mix together the mashed banana and shredded coconut. Then add coconut flour, chocolate chips, and stir well to cmbine.

• Shape the mixture into disks and set onto the baking sheet. Bake for twenty five minutes, until golden.

• Divide prepared cookies between meal prep containers and let cool down before storing in your fridge.

Sweet Energy Bites

Time: 15 mins

Number of servings: 10

Ingredients:

One cup old-fashioned rolled oats

Half cup pumpkin seeds

Quarter cup peanut butter

Four pitted dates

One Tbsp chia seeds

Half Tbsp raw honey

A pinch of cinnamon

Directions:

•	Place all your ingredients in your food processor and pulse for two minutes.

•	Divide the prepared mixture into ten parts and shape each into a ball.

•	Divide prepared sweet energy bites between meal prep containers and store in your fridge.

Multi-Seed Crackers

Time: 110 mins

Number of servings: 8

Ingredients:

Half cup raw sunflower seeds

Half cup sesame seeds

Half cup whole flaxseeds

Half cup ground flaxseeds

One tsp sesame seeds

One tsp poppy seeds

One tsp onion powder

One tsp garlic powder

One cup water

Directions:

• Place sunflower seeds in your food processor to break into smaller bits.

• In a large bowl, mix together all seeds, onion powder, garlic powder, and water. Stir well to combine and set aside for one hour to absorb water.

• Preheat your oven to 355°F and line a baking sheet with a parchment paper.

•	Now spread evenly prepared seed mixture on the lined baking sheet. Bake for thirty minutes, then let crackers sit in the oven for one hour.

•	Break up and divide prepared seed crackers between meal prep containers and store in your fridge.

Congratulations! No more looking in an open fridge trying to determine what to eat. Just grab your meal prep container and go!

Start small and prep only dinners for three days, for quick, easy, and healthy eating when you come home tired. Get good and fast at that, and then progress to adding lunches. However, you should avoid feeling overwhelmed. Don't go overboard at the start, and you will end up easily prepping breakfast, lunch, dinner, and snacks.

Add more flavor to your meals by using healthy sauces and spices. You can try a wide variety and choose your favorite. Limit consuming store-bought sauces because they contain excessive sugars, fat, sodium, and calories. Instead, whip up your own dressing or marinade with healthy ingredients like olive oil, lemon juice, grated ginger, onion, garlic, and herbs.

In order to achieve and maintain exceptional health and great shape, we need both healthy nutrition and physical activity. Naturally, your food planning should coincide with your fitness goals. Planning your workout routines and meals in the same notebook has a remarkable cross-fertilization effect!

I wish you to be healthy and happy!

Julia Schulte.

www.ingramcontent.com/pod-product-compliance
Lightning Source LLC
Chambersburg PA
CBHW081834250726
48659CB00008B/2451